DEDICATION

In memory of my parents, Elizabeth and Hans Sauer.
I would have loved to have shared this with you.

ABOUT THE AUTHOR

Author, columnist and media commentator Jost Sauer is a traditional Chinese medicine practitioner and lecturer. Apart from his own busy practice, Jost spends much of his year travelling, teaching and giving talks to the general public and health professionals. By continuing to examine ancient understandings about good health, then applying these insights to 21st-century issues, Jost has become one of the leading figures in innovative approaches to health and wellbeing.

Jost first came to attention with his groundbreaking books *Higher and Higher* and *Drug Repair That Works*. Passionate about good health, cars and electronic music, Jost offers his readers powerful, practical and effective new ways to approach the challenges of contemporary life.

CONTENTS

ACKNOWLEDGEMENTS

Foremost to my wife Kirsten, without whom this book would not exist. Elizabeth Stephens, editor of *Living Now*, for publishing a series of my articles on the chi cycle, and supporting my work in so many ways over the years. Maggie Hamilton, at Allen & Unwin, for continuing to believe in my vision. My father-in-law, Bryon Fitzpatrick, for once again providing support, stodge and storage space in the garage. Karina Averlon Thomas, for spreading the message and always encouraging me. Leon Fitzpatrick, for the enthusiastic feedback. To all my clients for giving me an opportunity to learn and grow.

Special thanks to the Chinese masters who have been refining the art of living for thousands of years. Without you I would have been a lost soul. I hope my contemporary interpretation of the chi cycle makes some small contribution to the ongoing evolution of this magical healing art.

Note on Traditional Chinese Medicine

In traditional Chinese medicine the word 'organs' refers to an organ system different to the anatomical system as understood in western medicine. It is convention to capitalise the name of an organ when referring to it in the Chinese context, but for ease of reading we are not applying this convention here. Likewise, we will not discuss pairs of organs in the singular.

Introduction

Traditional Chinese medicine is based on the idea that the universe is made of energy. This energy flows through the planets and stars, and also through our bodies, in a 24-hour cycle. In traditional Chinese medicine all life is interconnected and all things are possible.

Within our body, our life energy, or chi, circulates through each organ in turn. In traditional Chinese medicine we have twelve organs: the heart, small intestine, bladder, kidney, pericardium, san jiao (or triple burner), gall bladder, liver, lung, large intestine, stomach and spleen. 'Organ systems' is probably a better way to describe them as they also have meridians or invisible energy pathways associated with them. It is these pathways that allow energy to flow throughout our body and even extend beyond it.

Every two hours a different organ is energised. Each organ has a specific physical, emotional and spiritual function so every two hours there are certain things we should be doing to maximise the effect of the energised organ. This might be eating, working, exercising, meditating, having sex, sleeping or being creative. If we do the right things at the right time we don't waste our energy and we increase our longevity, happiness and health and take one step closer to fulfilling our destinies.

An organ's pathways can also access what is known as the universal intelligence, a source of great wisdom. So, every two hours a different part of life's wisdom is available to us. For example, each day between 1 and 3 pm, as our small intestine is energised, we have an opportunity to find mental clarity. Between 3 and 5 pm, as our bladder becomes energised, we can feel our direct connection to life. If we don't accept these gifts at the time, life simply offers them again the next day.

Another great thing about this cycle—which we will refer to as the chi cycle or Perfect Day Plan—is that regardless of how depressed, lethargic or ill we might feel, every day we have an opportunity to change. All we have to do is get our actions in tune with the cycle and our health will automatically improve. Each thing we do at the right time with one organ makes it easier for the next organ to carry out its duties, which in turn impacts on how the day ahead pans out physically, emotionally and spiritually.

A key element of the Perfect Day Plan is balancing action (yang) times with rest (yin) times. This is a huge challenge for our current lifestyle of 24/7 activity. We all know we can't keep this up, but at the same time it seems impossible to stop—we don't seem to have enough time to get things done. The chi cycle shows the optimum times to take breaks so that the active times are much more effective and productive—the Perfect Day Plan gives time back to us.

This plan works. I've turned my life around by living it, and so have countless clients and workshop participants and it is easy to do. Following the Perfect Day Plan is not about giving up things, it is about doing things at the appropriate times so we don't lose vital life energy and end up with digestive problems, chronic fatigue, food allergies, road rage, addiction, psychosis, obesity, heart disease and panic disorders.

Parents often say they wished their children came with instructions . . . in fact we do. The chi cycle maps out everything for us. It was identified thousands of years ago by the ancient Chinese sages, but right now we are probably entering the first time in history where we can actually live it. After centuries of restraint and control, we can now choose *how* we want to live. We can choose the chi cycle lifestyle. We can follow the Perfect Day Plan.

Chapter 1

Your Perfect Day Plan

What if you were able to unlock the secret to making every day work for you? What if you knew the best time to eat and sleep, to exercise and to chill out, when to do your most demanding work, the ideal time to let go of the past, when you're most likely to come up with good ideas, and all the other things that would make life easier?

The great news is that the map for your perfect day already exists. Over thousands of years Chinese sages have not only discovered how our organs work, but how each of them impacts on our emotions and spirit. So, if an organ isn't functioning as it should be, it not only affects your physical wellbeing but how you relate to yourself and others on an emotional level. And, because mind, body and spirit are linked, it also has an impact on your spirit.

This ancient health plan really works and it is simple to follow. For two hours each day, each organ has its time in the sun. Once you understand the basics you will know the best time to do certain things and avoid others depending on which organ's time it is. You will know how to nurture yourself through your lifestyle so that you get a head-start not only every day but also on life.

In the Perfect Day Plan each organ has an area of influence. For example, on a physical level your kidneys are connected with your sex drive, so if you are losing interest in sex and then having issues with your partner it could be a kidney issue rather than a relationship issue. The Perfect Day Plan helps you understand why you are feeling or reacting the way you are and what you need to do to sort out your imbalances. It really helps to know that when you are feeling anxious, experiencing panic attacks, chronic fatigue or depression that certain organs are in need of attention.

The Perfect Day Plan is not about rigidly sticking to a system and obsessing about what to do every two hours— there are many situations or circumstances beyond our control. But the great thing is once we get enough perfect days under our belts we start to feel good—really good— and the way we should feel. Then, when we deviate from the cycle, we immediately understand why we don't feel right the next day and we know how to correct it.

Being able to self-correct means you don't have to go to a doctor with a host of seemingly inexplicable symptoms of 'not feeling right', of tiredness, depression and exhaustion that will invite antidepressants or other medications.

In a few simple steps this straightforward plan teaches you how to nourish each organ. And when you do this you discover that it impacts on all your other organs, until everything is in balance. By capturing the momentum each two-hour period offers, the Perfect Day Plan helps you make the most of each day. So instead of feeling as if everything is hard work, you are able to be the energised, motivated upbeat person you'd like to be.

We want to be awake to ourselves and make the most of every opportunity. So, let's get into a 24-hour cycle and see exactly what we need to do to achieve all we were destined to.

Chapter 2

Getting Some Balance

7 am to 9 am

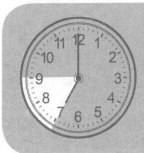

BODY PART – STOMACH

KEY THOUGHT – ARRIVE

TIME TO . . .

Be sweet to yourself, eat breakfast, feel balance

WELCOME TO EARTH

The chi cycle is continuous, it doesn't really start or finish anywhere, but I'm going to kick off with 7 am to 9 am because there is one simple thing that you can do in these two hours that will make immediate positive changes in your life.

It is also a good place to begin because in Chinese medicine 7 am is the time of the earth element. All our organs are associated with one of the five elements— water, wood, fire, earth and metal—and each has different qualities. The earth element is all about being grounded and solid.

You could think of yourself at this time each morning as being welcomed to earth. It's an opportunity to get in touch with your body before you launch into emails, phone calls, work and other exciting activities that take us out of our bodies and into our heads.

DELAY THE HIT

Between 7 and 9 am our energy is in our stomach and the most important thing to do is have breakfast. Lots of people stumble out of bed and head straight for a cup of coffee or tea, but this speeds us up and launches us into the day without giving ourselves the chance to enjoy a bit of quality time in the earth element.

I am not saying give up your morning coffee, only delay it. Living in harmony with the Perfect Day Plan is all about shifting things. If you are a first-up coffee or tea drinker, try and hold off until after breakfast. These drinks interfere with your appetite and, as we are about to find out, you don't want anything doing this.

A TASTE FOR LIFE

In traditional Chinese medicine our taste for life comes from our stomach, so by eating the right breakfast with the right attitude we will naturally want to sample everything life has to offer. We will be adventurous, lively, engaged and balanced people—everyone will want to be our friend.

Our taste for life comes from our stomach, so by eating the right breakfast with the right attitude we will naturally want to sample everything life has to offer. We will be adventurous, lively, engaged and balanced.

Eating breakfast is essential to our health and happiness but somewhere along the way it dropped off our 'to do' list. The majority of my clients say 'I don't eat breakfast', as if it's optional or irrelevant. It isn't. We all have to eat breakfast, it's a necessity. If we skip breakfast and other meals it reduces our taste for life. It also contributes to the inability to get out of bed in the morning, and to weak limbs, loose stools, loss of appetite and even mental confusion.

Life and Death and Breakfast

Eating a good breakfast builds stomach chi or energy. This is really important. It is said 'If there

Eating a good breakfast builds stomach chi or energy.

is stomach chi there is life, if there is no stomach chi there is death'. So eating a good breakfast really is a life and death matter! If you regularly skip breakfast you will deplete your stomach chi. Then your body will weaken, you won't be able to bounce back from illnesses and you will be more prone to anxiety, panic attacks, chronic fatigue and depression. Of course most people never connect these symptoms with skipping breakfast. They start feeling emotionally down and, thinking they have a chemical imbalance in the brain, head off to get antidepressants or other powerful medications. Before they know it they are living an unhappy, uncomfortable and medicated life.

You can help avoid this simply by always eating a nice warm breakfast. The warm part is important. Fresh fruit may seem like a good healthy breakfast, but it doesn't build strong stomach energy. No cold or raw food does because your body has to use up your precious energy to 'cook' it. Imagine your stomach as a big empty pot with a small flame under it. If you put a whole lot of cold, uncooked things in the pot it's going to take a really long time to cook and you will use a lot of fuel. Not only that, cold food is a shock to the stomach, so after a cold breakfast we will feel unsettled and emotionally unstable for the day.

If you warm up your food first it will take a lot less of your fuel. It will also help build energy and improve your health and longevity. Do yourself a favour and have your fruit in the afternoon as a snack (if you need one) and start your day with a warm, cooked breakfast.

Be Sweet to Yourself

The taste of earth is sweet, so you want to have 'sweet' cereals for breakfast. By this I mean things like oats, not breakfast cereals full of sugar. Processed cereals are very appealing in the morning because, as we are in the time of the earth element, we intuitively seek sweetness but sugary cereals only create an impression of pleasure by using up our life energy. At stomach time we should be sweet to ourselves and eat food that provides emotional support.

Everyone's diet is different but generally speaking a porridge or congee of cooked oats or rice, barley, millet or buckwheat is a good choice. Oatmeal porridge is my favourite. Organic oat porridge can balance emotional levels in the body and it's great for building your taste for life. Toast is not a chi building food but, if you love toast for breakfast, try and make it a rye or other non-wheat bread. Eating wheat in the morning makes you feel tired and that is the wrong way to start a perfect day. It can kick off what I call a 'reverse cycle' day, where everything you do is compensating for the last thing. You eat toast for breakfast, you

> Eating wheat in the morning makes you feel tired and that is the wrong way to start a perfect day.

feel exhausted by 10 am, you need coffee and cake to keep going, and you end up using all your energy rather than building it. A run of reverse cycle days can start off a reverse cycle life and none of us want this.

Can't Face Breakfast?

If you regularly skip breakfast and other meals you lose your appetite because your organs, particularly your spleen, become deficient and don't function properly. A lifestyle of over-study, over-work and over-worry contributes to this as well.

If you can't face breakfast, don't try and force down a big bowl of porridge. Start off by building up your energy by taking protein powder, supplements and Chinese raw herbs. These are very nutritious but easily digestible. Then you can try and eat small portions of warm cooked foods and build up to eating larger meals. Get some acupuncture too to help build up your chi.

ALCOHOL AND THE STOMACH

Denise was a client of mine who got caught in the reverse cycle lifestyle and ended up as an 'alcoholic'. The first thing I did was ask her about her diet. She was around fifty and said it had been thirty years since she last ate breakfast. Lunch was toasted cheese sandwiches at her desk. These do not build life energy. Her dinner was salad or takeaway food. As a result of this nutrient-deprived diet her stomach and other organs could not function properly, she was permanently ungrounded, exhausted and confused, and she needed a couple of bottles of wine to get to sleep at night. Thinking she was an alcoholic, she went to daily meetings where the idea of addiction was constantly reinforced.

I immediately started Denise on powerful nutritional supplements, improved her diet, introduced some chi-cycle-friendly activities and eventually she lost her need for alcohol. Now Denise is in charge of her life and has an occasional drink when she feels like it.

I do not believe addiction is a disease. It is a side effect of not knowing about the chi cycle. I have treated plenty of so-called alcoholics who would have one drink then couldn't stop. But once they got into a different way of living, getting drunk lost its appeal. If you follow the Perfect Day Plan, it makes you powerful over all substances.

GOING TO GROUND

After one of my recent talks on the chi cycle, someone asked if there was something 'colder' than porridge she could eat in the morning. If you want cold foods for breakfast, or any other time, it is possibly because you have what we call a 'heat condition' and are subconsciously seeking to balance this. Heat symptoms include frustration, anger, itchy skin, mood swings, sexual voraciousness and insomnia, and you might feel physically hot. Chinese raw herbs are fantastic for alleviating these, but eating cold foods can actually make things worse. So try and avoid cold foods any time, but especially in the morning, even if you do crave them.

Our stomach energy (chi) grounds us. It gives us deep roots in our life.

Other clients tell me they can't eat porridge because it makes them feel tired or heavy. Our stomach energy (chi) grounds us. It gives us deep roots in our life. A warm porridge for breakfast allows you to feel this but if you are depleted and weak or have too much of what we call 'yang', the grounding action of the stomach can feel like tiredness and heaviness. This feeling can make people want to skip breakfast but that is not the answer; seeking balance by following the Perfect Day Plan and living the chi cycle and building your energy and appetite for life is.

Even if you don't have any imbalances but still have difficulty eating porridge, the second best option is something like buckwheat pancakes, so you could try them for a while. Once you get other chi cycle activities in place your appetite will pick up. Eventually you will start craving nourishing foods like porridge. What you are craving though is not the porridge itself, but the way it makes you feel grounded and simultaneously energetic. This is much better than a frenetic caffeine energy rush and it increases, rather than reduces, your taste for life.

You will start craving nourishing foods like porridge. What you are craving though is not the porridge itself, but the way it makes you feel grounded and simultaneously energetic.

Jost's Porridge Recipe
serves 2

Ingredients

1 cup organic oats
¾ litre to 1 litre soy or oat milk (you can also use cow's milk)
2 to 3 tablespoons poppy seeds
1 teaspoon ginger
1 tablespoon organic honey
3 tablespoons protein powder (I use a whey protein isolate)
dash cinnamon

Method

Put the oats, milk and a handful of poppy seeds in a pot the evening before, and leave in the fridge so that the oats can soak overnight. The following morning, put the pot on the stove on a low heat and let it slowly come to the boil. Allow to simmer for 5 minutes, turn the heat off and let it cool slightly. Add the ginger, honey, protein powder and cinnamon. Mix well. Remember that everything is chi (energy), including porridge, so cook with the intention of building your energy and appetite for life.

Jost's Buckweat Pancakes

serves 4

Ingredients

1 cup buckwheat flour (you can also use maize—a corn flour)

1 cup gluten-free SR flour (I use one which is a mix of rice and potato)

handful oats

2 eggs

1 tablespoon oil

1¾ cup soy milk

Method

Sift the flours into a bowl, then add the oats. Beat the eggs lightly, add the oil and pour the mixture into the bowl. Add the soy milk (if the mixture is too thick, add extra milk). Mix well and let stand for 30 minutes. Then place spoonfuls of the mix into a hot frying pan. Turn when bubbles appear to brown on other side. Top with organic honey.

WHEN YOU HAVE NO TASTE

At one stage I treated Susan, a middle-aged woman who had lost her sense of taste. She said she might as well have been eating cardboard. Susan was working in a male-dominated scientific field and always felt she had to work twice as hard as her colleagues to prove herself. She got up at six, drank a couple of coffees and went to work. Sometimes she ate a muffin for morning tea at her desk. She never ate breakfast, rarely had time for lunch and usually worked until seven each night. She then took work home and heated up frozen meals for dinner. She said she had to do this because otherwise she would never get on top of her work.

Funnily enough, for someone who rarely ate, Susan's greatest pleasure in life was cooking. On Sundays she would spend the morning shopping for exotic ingredients and then prepare a gourmet lunch for her husband and their friends. She was devastated when she could no longer taste anything. Susan went to specialists who tried everything they could think of, but nothing changed. Eventually she decided to look at alternative medicine and came to see me. After assessing her lifestyle, diet and the health of her organs, the solution was clear. She had severely depleted stomach and spleen chi, and had to immediately change her eating and work habits.

Susan was highly sceptical. Specialists had been presenting her with complex medical theories so having a nice cooked breakfast, regular meals and taking some time away from her desk sounded overly simplistic. She tried it though and, combined with acupuncture and Chinese raw herbs, her taste started coming back within weeks. Some things in life are that simple.

GETTING THE MESSAGE

Our organs have physical, emotional and spiritual properties so you can look at imbalances and illnesses as having a special message for a patient.

Our organs have physical, emotional and spiritual properties in traditional Chinese medicine, so you can look at imbalances and illnesses as having a special message for a patient. In Susan's case, she had depleted her stomach energy and lost her taste for food. Food equals life, so it was a message for her that if she didn't change she would lose her taste for living. We are such a rational society we have forgotten that we are a part of the universe and that it offers us support in many ways. We see our illnesses as problems and medicate them into oblivion. We miss the chance to understand the incredible potential of our organs to teach us how to live the kind of life we dream of.

THE ART OF EATING

I treat a lot of clients who have forgotten they have to eat, but also a lot of clients who have forgotten *how* to eat. We commonly stuff down meals in front of the TV, digesting bad news and depressing images at the same time. Or we eat on the way to work, while walking around the shopping centre or standing up in the kitchen and doing other things. How to eat is as important as what to eat. Stomach energy 'descends'—it sends food downwards so your body can use the nutrients. Watching TV, reading the paper, answering the phone or sending texts or emails are 'yang' activities that drive your energy upwards. If you do those

> Watching TV, reading the paper, answering the phone or sending texts or emails are 'yang' activities that drive your energy upwards. If you do those things while you eat, only a small percentage of the nutrients in your food will end up being absorbed.

things while you eat, only a small percentage of the nutrients in your food will end up being absorbed.

Sit down to eat, straighten your back, shake your neck loose and try to let your shoulders relax. Because we are all so busy we unconsciously hunch our shoulders but this makes it harder to digest properly, which lays the foundation for irritable bowel syndrome and other digestive disorders. Before each mouthful think 'down' or 'I'm here now'. As you chew, visualise a force pulling your food down. Be in your body, feel its weight, feel the pull of the earth.

Be silent and eat in peace. Because food creates life, if we eat while stressed or running over old arguments in our head it turns our food against us and cements those negative emotions in our bowels. At stomach time it is all about what is happening in our internal world. We don't want to know what is happening in the outside world yet. So save watching the news until later. At stomach time, the only thing that matters is the here and now.

Arrival Lounge

The focus is on being slow. If you can work towards giving yourself at least ten (ideally twenty) peaceful minutes to sit and eat breakfast somewhere between 7 and 9 am, you will start to get the fantastic feeling of being energised and calm at the same time. I call this having 'arrived'. It is a gift on offer for us at stomach time. It's worth getting up ten minutes earlier to give yourself some extra time to eat, just to get a glimpse of this.

If you go to see a spiritual teacher, you can get a taste of 'arrival' simply by being in their presence. A post-orgasm glow can, to a lesser degree, be the same. Achieving this state in the morning while we eat is our goal for stomach time.

Departure Time

Arrival is a result of balance and it is becoming a rare experience in our action-based yang culture. I once had the opportunity to meet a famous success guru but by the time he shook my hand he had already moved on to the next thing in his head. After meeting him I realised he was a master of departure and most of us are on a similar path. We are on to the next thing before we have even finished what we are currently doing. Many people gulp down breakfast while already thinking about work. Eating like this erodes health and happiness. We have to train ourselves to eat while consciously being in our bodies.

SUCCESS AND THE STOMACH

If we don't ever get the feeling of having arrived it contributes to that constant niggling sense that something is missing in life. This is fuelling the new plague of unhappiness sweeping across society and is contributing to the boom in success seminars and publications. Generally speaking, these only offer a solution to our unhappiness or dissatisfaction through strategies to achieve material success. Those they attract want things to be different but often end up more dissatisfied with life. This is because there is also a *physical* aspect to success and it is connected with strong stomach chi.

I treat many mid-life crisis clients who have achieved all their business goals and gained great wealth but are not healthy or happy. Material success alone doesn't make you happy. Don't get me wrong here, I'm not against the idea. I love hot cars, recording equipment and technological gadgets, but you need a good set of organs and strong stomach chi to enjoy your success.

You can still have success if you don't have healthy organs, but it will be success built on a weak foundation and destined to collapse. By eating a warm, nourishing breakfast in a peaceful environment we build stomach energy. A person with strong stomach energy is powerful, but soft and gentle as well. He or she can wait, but they have the power to act instantly. They feel balance in action and rest, so they naturally attract success.

> A person with strong stomach energy is powerful, but soft and gentle as well. They feel balance in action and rest, so they naturally attract success.

BALANCE AND THE STOMACH

Many success gurus don't have a balance between action (yang) and rest (yin). They have what we call a strong yang constitution. They are extroverts who have a really high sex drive and can appear totally inconsiderate of the opinions of others. For them it is harder not to do something than to do it. On stage they can inspire an audience solely by their excess of yang energy. Their recommendations, such as eating raw foods or only eating fruit until lunchtime, are often based on their constitutional type rather than universal truths. But if they do not build their yin to an equal level sooner or later they will crash.

In traditional Chinese medicine we also have the opposite, the totally yin types who are too shy to voice an opinion or put anyone out. These people have a much lower sex drive and need more sleep than the yang types. They easily get drunk, are more prone to paranoia and were often sickly as a child. They find it harder to do something than not to do it. Eating raw foods or nothing but fruit until lunchtime for this type of people is highly detrimental. They need a different diet and lifestyle to feel successful.

Both yin and yang types have their advantages and disadvantages. Most of us are somewhere in between. Between 7 and 9 am,

> Between 7 and 9 am is the most important time for us to address our imbalances because our stomach is supporting actions that create balance.

however, is the most important time for us to address our imbalances because our stomach is supporting actions that create balance. You might be an active yang type, but have developed deficient organs due to an inappropriate lifestyle. This means you have all the ideas and drive of your yang nature, but are no longer able to follow through. This is incredibly frustrating. What and how you eat in stomach time can help change this.

TIME AND THE STOMACH

When I suggest spending ten or fifteen minutes in the morning on a peaceful breakfast, many clients immediately say they don't have the time for that. But time is relative. If you want to see time slow down, get on a treadmill, set the timer for thirty minutes and start running really hard. One minute stretches to eternity!

In traditional Chinese medicine our perception of time is regulated by our organs, and the relationship between yin and yang. If yin is in excess, time slows down. If yang is in excess, everything speeds up. As we are rushing through life and racing through breakfast we are losing our yin skills and experiencing a yang spike. As a result, we feel we have less and less time. Our stomach plays an important role in

Taking the time to eat a good breakfast in the right conditions *creates* time. It allows us to feel time is with us, not against us.

changing this. Taking the time to eat a good breakfast in the right conditions *creates* time. It allows us to feel time is with us, not against us.

The solution to our 'lack of time' and 'never catching up' lies in learning to live in harmony with the chi cycle and in learning to 'arrive' during breakfast. You will feel on top of things all day and won't end up caught on the wheel working harder and harder, trying to get everything under control. You will get a free ticket to escape the rat race.

Between 7 and 9 am, remind yourself that you are being welcomed to earth. Spend your fifteen minutes of breakfast time trying to get in touch with your stomach chi. Then, on your way to work or as you go about your business until 9 am, maybe listen to music or CDs that zone you into the now. What you want to reinforce at this time in the morning is the sense that, ultimately, 'nothing matters'. This is a powerful yin concept and it puts you in the right physical and emotional place to start a perfect day.

Chapter 3
Action Time

9 am to 11 am

BODY PART – SPLEEN
KEY THOUGHT – ACTION
TIME TO . . .
Work hard, think, do

GO, GO, GO

By 9 am our inner energy (chi) has spent two hours in our stomach and it now moves to our spleen. If you allowed yourself to *arrive* by eating a warm, nutritious breakfast in a nice peaceful environment during stomach time (7 to 9 am), you are now fuelled up and ready to power through the morning.

In spleen time you are being offered an opportunity to get behind the wheel, open up the throttle and see what you've got under the hood. You have full support for this now from your spleen, but also from the universal energy source, so don't hold back. This is the time of day to make the most of our speedy yang natures by really going for it.

Eating slowly and thinking about 'now' during stomach time allowed you to build some yin qualities (yin is downward motion). Now, in spleen time, our energy is on the up. So in these two hours all your thoughts and actions are going to be aligned with an upward force. This means that for the next few hours you have full support for action. This is the time to get out your 'to do' list and start crossing off items.

Study Hard

Between 9 and 11 am is the best time to concentrate and memorise information. You will absorb and recall what you read or listen to. Most students study at night because there is less going on around them, which creates the impression that they can focus better and learn more. But it is the worst time for this as it will force you to draw on inner energy resources. In the evening your energy has moved into different organs and you are supposed to be nurturing your soul or relaxing, not giving your brain a workout.

WHERE WAS I?

Our spleen is responsible for carrying our thoughts around. When you start forgetting things halfway through a sentence you know your spleen doesn't have the chi it needs to operate properly. You need to nurture your spleen by living in harmony with the chi cycle, because once your spleen does not have enough energy or chi you lose your boundaries, forget what you are saying and become confused and paranoid. It is very unpleasant.

> When you start forgetting things halfway through a sentence you know your spleen doesn't have the chi it needs to operate properly.

TIME TO TALK

If the spleen has plenty of energy, 9 to 11 am is a positive time. The spleen smoothes out emotions. In fact, it is the least emotionally reactive time of the day. This makes between 9 and 11 am the perfect time to deal with difficult people and problems. Make the most of this two-hour window to see your most taxing clients, talk about who takes the garbage out, ask your boss for a raise, discuss sensitive matters or phone that person you have been meaning to apologise to. It is also the best time to tackle relationship issues. If you want to have a serious discussion with your partner or spouse do it over a cup of tea mid-morning, not in the evening after work and never, ever over drinks late at night (this is the most emotionally reactive time of the chi cycle). You should save potentially emotional discussions for mid-morning because, as long as your spleen is healthy, you will have the support to resolve things. If your spleen is not healthy, don't even go there. Conversations will go round in circles and get nowhere or make things worse.

MIS-TREATS

The middle of spleen time is when most people have their morning tea. I'm not a great fan of the idea as the stomach is a large muscle which is supposed to expand and contract a few times a day. After the fullness of breakfast it needs some emptiness. You want to give your stomach three decent meals a day, not lots of snacks. Constant grazing leads to all kinds of spleen imbalances. It can cause a short attention span and a lack of focus and patience so you can be easily aggravated.

Many chefs suffer from this. Everything is fine, they are whistling over their stock pot, then a second later they are throwing fish at people's heads. Their shifts don't allow regular meals, so they snack instead. Or, because they are constantly tasting as they cook, their appetite is reduced. Nibbling becomes more appealing than eating a proper meal and this takes a toll on the organs and leads to mood swings.

Constant grazing leads to all kinds of spleen imbalances. It can cause a short attention span and a lack of focus and patience so you can be easily aggravated.

Six Small Meals

There are plenty of theories about eating six small meals a day but that type of diet is designed to stabilise emotions, so it comes from a starting point of instability or imbalance. If you eat three proper meals a day, take supplements and live in harmony with the Perfect Day Plan, your emotions will automatically be stable. A breakfast of a good nutritious porridge (with protein powder added in) will support you for four hours. Lunch should support you for six hours—especially if you take nutritional supplements as well. Lots of people think if they eat well they won't need extra vitamins and minerals, but the simple truth is we can no longer function properly without supplements. Even if we eat only healthy food it is just not nutritious enough any more. If it was, none of us would need snacks at any time of the day. Snacking emerged as the quality of our food declined.

Tea and Pumpkin

Cakes and biscuits for morning tea emerged as we forgot how to live and people started running out of energy by mid-morning. If you do need something at this time of day, I would recommend a nice cup of green tea and perhaps something savoury, rather than sweet biscuits or cakes. Between 9 and 11 am we are still in the earth element and, like the stomach, the spleen loves sweetness. Pumpkin is a classic sweet spleen food, but we don't think of some steamed pumpkin for morning tea, we think of sugar.

> If you need something at this time of day, I recommend a nice cup of green tea and something savoury, rather than sweet biscuits or cakes.

Our relationship with sugar needs a major overhaul. It is thought of as a treat, a reward, or something to cheer ourselves up. But you will come down from a sugar high and then you will feel worse. If you are feeling depressed,

> If you are feeling depressed, lethargic or unhappy, the best thing you can do for yourself is get physically fit

lethargic or unhappy, the best thing you can do for yourself is get a six-pack. By this I don't mean beer but stomach muscles. Being physically fit and in tune with the chi cycle is the most powerful antidepressant on earth.

The Feast Day

We don't have to be rigid about following the Perfect Day Plan. I suggest keeping what I call a 'feast day' in each week where you break all the rules. If you do want to eat something sweet, have it around four in the afternoon on your feast day when you can afford to feel tired afterwards, then lie around and do nothing. Having a feast day to look forward to also encourages you to stay in tune with the plan during the week.

GO AHEAD, MAKE MY DAY

All our organs work in pairs and between 9 and 11 am our spleen is working in conjunction with its partner the stomach. The stomach gathers food, the spleen converts it. You could say the spleen 'makes your day' because it takes everything you have been thinking, eating and doing so far and converts this into your energy for the day. If you have been living in accord with the chi cycle, it has the nutrients from your warm, cooked breakfast that you ate in peace and your feeling of having arrived from stomach time to work with. It takes all this up to your heart, where it is turned into blood and love. With this material to work with, it can make you a beautiful day.

If you follow the thoughts and actions of the chi cycle every day, it will build the foundation for a beautiful life. But if you are on the reverse cycle and sleep in, wake up hating the day ahead, drag yourself out of bed, turn on the TV, slurp coffee while puffing on a ciggie and driving to work then have fast food at your desk, the spleen only has a pile of toxic thoughts and actions to work with. It can only make more of the same for your day ahead. Making a day is the same as making a meal: it is only as good as the ingredients. This is why it is so crucial to put in a big effort to get the first few hours of the day right. If we don't it can lead to ill-health and a life full of unresolved issues.

> Making a day is the same as making a meal: it is only as good as the ingredients.

IBS AND THE SPLEEN

Patricia was a 34-year-old journalist who suffered from irritable bowel syndrome. She had alternating constipation then explosive diarrhoea, which she couldn't afford in her line of work, so she ended up medicated. The drugs made her feel sick so she wanted to explore other options. From waking, Patricia allowed herself 17 minutes to get to work.

She had no breakfast, rushed around madly answering the phone, dealing with her kids and husband, then sped off anticipating the dramas of the day ahead.

By eight she was at her desk reading reports and looking at graphic images of all the terrible things that had happened overnight. Then, before she had a chance to even grab a cup of tea, she would usually rush out to a site of death and destruction. Desperate to get there before the opposition, she would throw some sandwiches in the car and nibble at the red lights while anticipating the gory scene ahead.

All Patricia had given her spleen to work with was stress, fast food and terrible thoughts and images. Because she drove herself so hard to stay on top of her home and work life, she was all about control and no surrender. There was no balance of yin and yang and this interfered with the upwards and downwards flow of her chi. Instead of nutrients and positive thoughts going up to the heart and waste products moving down to be eliminated, it was as if the opposite was happening. This created constant irritation in Patricia's system, resulting in an irritable bowel.

To avoid digestive problems, fatigue, dizziness, an impaired sense of taste, prolapsed organs, poor memory, dull thinking and lack of concentration, get in sync with the chi cycle and give the stomach and spleen what they need to function properly.

Get in sync with the chi cycle and give the stomach and spleen what they need to function properly.

THE TUBE BODY

Your spleen impacts on the shape of your body. If your spleen is healthy it will transform fluids and you will have shapely muscles and a well-toned body. If your spleen is deficient you will have fluid retention, pale skin, no muscle tone and flab around the hips.

A lot of people are now developing a 'tube body', one with no waist. Some suggest this is physical evolution but I see it as an imbalance of the spleen. By nature we have a waist and it has a purpose. It is here that the girdle channel, the only circular energy pathway in the body, regulates the upward and downward movement of energy. If this movement is impaired, due to incorrect food and lifestyle, fat accumulates around the waist and hips.

The tube body is becoming very common now, especially among the younger generation, as a result of eating processed, nutrient-deprived foods and too much sugar. We want to avoid this because the impaired energy flow can lead to serious imbalances. We want the perfect body with all our organs in perfect working order, and that comes from living in harmony with natural forces.

Chapter 4
Express Yourself
11 am to 1 pm

BODY PART – HEART
KEY THOUGHT – LOVE
TIME TO . . .
Work smart, access your soul,
spread the love

SATISFY YOUR SOUL

Every two hours, as a new organ becomes charged with life energy, it is as if we are also being offered a glimpse into the amazing nature of our inner world. At eleven in the morning our chi moves to our heart and the next two hours are all about purpose and joy.

In traditional Chinese medicine the heart is very special.

The ancient texts refer to it as the sun or the emperor and the other organs make offerings to it and protect it. It is the seat of our consciousness and intelligence and governs our body. It is also the home of our soul. This means between 11 am and 1 pm, when our life energy is in our heart, we are able to get in touch with our soul and have an opportunity to find purpose in our life.

SPREAD THE LOVE

Our heart communicates ideas; it sends our thoughts out. At 11 am we have moved from the earth to the fire element, and at heart time our thoughts can spread like flames. This means that between 11 am and 1 pm we are at our most expressive. If you are in business make the most of this by scheduling inspirational meetings

> Between 11 am and 1 pm we are at our most expressive.

with colleagues or people who assist you in realising your creative ideas. This is also the best time to make really important work decisions, so schedule your board meetings for this time too.

If you have a mindless job or a job that you hate, try and spend some time between 11 am and 1 pm thinking about what *you* want to do. Imagine yourself going back to college or pursuing your dream career. What feels right for you at this time will be connected with your destiny and purpose in life. If you are a student, this makes heart time ideal for planning your studies.

Wherever you are, try and keep meaning, intelligence and soul in mind in these two hours. Engage with this on some level. This could be by writing a journal entry about what you want to do in life, or speaking to people about what is closest to your heart and who you really are. It is also a good time to set spiritual goals and to seek out people who will help, inspire and encourage you on that path. The universal energy supports this and the fire element will spread your aspirations, helping to attract what you want. Heart time is a beautiful part of the day.

VISITING THE EMPEROR

I like to think of heart time as an opportunity to have an 'audience with the emperor'. The idea is to save up the really important and meaningful things to put on the table in this meeting.

I treat many clients who spend their heart time watching TV. Sitting back watching soapies or talk shows or doing things that aren't concerned with your purpose in life at heart time means turning down the opportunity to find meaning, and joy drains out of your life. I'm not saying don't watch TV, rather don't watch TV when you have a chance to get in touch with what is closest to your soul. Record your favourite shows then watch them somewhere between

5 and 9 pm when your energy is in other organs and you are supposed to be entertaining yourself and relaxing.

GET SMART

In each 24-hour cycle the energetic forces of the universe slowly shift from yang (action) to yin (rest). The yang phase starts at midnight and peaks at noon. This is followed by a yin phase which slowly builds until it peaks at midnight. Right in the middle of heart time we hit noon, the most yang time of the entire cycle. This is when the fire is burning brightest and we are at our most alert.

> At work, we need to be highly productive, but we want to work smarter rather than harder.

At work, to make the most of this yang peak, we need to be highly productive, but we want to work smarter rather than harder. Working hard belongs in the preceding hours of spleen time. As our spleen belongs to the earth element there is a 'weight' to our actions then. There is effort involved in getting things done and you can feel it. But we are now in the fire element and fire spreads effortlessly. The idea is to push yourself between 9 and 11 am to build momentum, and then between 11 am and 1 pm to be really productive intellectually knowing that, as things shift from yang to yin on a universal level, you have an opportunity to tap into that universal momentum to help you through the rest of the day.

WHO ARE YOU?

As well as communicating our ideas, our heart communicates who we are to the world. You can either come across as a loving, calm and centred person who inspires those around you, or a depressed, angry, negative and needy person whom others avoid. These are not personality types or disorders—there is no such thing in traditional Chinese medicine. The way you behave is simply the outcome of how closely you live in accordance with the chi cycle and how much you nourish your organs and your heart. We all want to be loving, calm and happy people. All we have to do is focus on living the chi cycle, and build up our chi and our blood.

Our heart communicates who we are to the world. You can either come across as a loving, calm and centred person who inspires those around you, or a depressed, angry, negative and needy person whom others avoid.

THE STOCK POT

In traditional Chinese medicine blood is a magical elixir of life. It provides the basis for our thoughts and our wellbeing. If we imagine our blood as a chef's stock simmering away on the stove, we want to be constantly adding good things to it to make a rich, 'hearty' broth. If we live by the Perfect

Day Plan we are off to a good start because we begin the day by putting in lots of energy and nutrients from our warm nourishing breakfast, and then add the power of our hard work at spleen time. If we do this regularly and add in all the other wonderful gifts of the day such as wisdom, clarity of thought and courage, it will create a truly life-changing potion. At eleven each morning, as our chi energises our heart and blood production reaches a peak, our heart will have all the ingredients it needs for creating joy and peace within us and around us.

The trick is to keep in mind that everything that goes into our stock pot either improves our broth or contaminates it. If we have too much junk food or too many negative thoughts and live a reverse cycle life, our blood will be weak. Instead of feeling joyous we are headed for depression.

DEPRESSION AND THE HEART

I recently treated Tony, a 45-year-old businessman who ran a huge construction company. He was very successful and had everything he thought he had ever wanted. Cars were his passion and he had finally achieved his goal of owning a Ferrari. But Tony was overweight, had hypertension, was on blood-pressure medication and sleeping pills and was depressed. He resented the business he used to love and couldn't enjoy the car he had worked so hard for. He knew he needed to change but didn't know how and had no energy or motivation to find out.

I asked Tony what he wanted in life and he said to go back to the 'good old days', to the fun and excitement he felt when he was young. He had tried going to bars where young people hung out, but just felt more depressed. He was on the right track, just going about it the wrong way. He needed to recapture the good old days, but a lot of what made them so good were healthy organs. If we keep up our chi and blood maintenance and live by the Perfect Day Plan, every day can be a 'good old day'. Our lungs will have lots of energy and allow us to embrace change, let go of the past and envision an exciting future. Our liver keeps the energy flowing smoothly so we feel happy. Our spleen gives us boundaries and makes us want to communicate with people. Our kidneys give us the power to face our fears and do things. Our heart spreads love, inspiration and joy. If you put all this together you produce the opposite state to depression.

Antidepressants: The New Gateway Drug

In traditional Chinese medicine, depression is all about how you live and the state of your organs, blood and chi. Antidepressants are not the solution. They might hold off your symptoms for

In traditional Chinese medicine, depression is all about how you live and the state of your organs, blood and chi.

a while, but eventually (like recreational drugs) anti-depressants increase organ deficiencies. Not only that but they are fast becoming a new gateway drug. I am starting to see a lot of clients who are addicted to speed or ice but when I ask them when they had their first joint, as this is generally how people start a drug journey, they look at me blankly. These clients never used recreational drugs, but were prescribed antidepressants. As their antidepressants stopped working they tried others, then shifted to speed or ice.

Depression has a physiological base. Medication and partying aren't the solution. The path forward is to follow the Perfect Day Plan, take up the chi cycle lifestyle, build up your energy and nourish your blood so your organs can operate properly again. Tony had been doing the opposite. He ate takeaway on the run, had insomnia, did not exercise, lived in a state of stress and medicated himself so he could keep functioning. He still took loving care of his Ferrari though. I asked if he ever put low-grade fuel in its tank and took it off-road on the weekend. He looked so shocked it was almost comical. I suggested he think of himself as a luxury vehicle, which meant he too needed high-grade fuel, or healthy blood and chi, to keep his engine maintained and reach his peak performance. At present his lifestyle was the equivalent of bush-bashing a Ferrari.

If Tony committed to building his inner health the way he had committed to building his business, he would start to enjoy his life and success again. The first step for him was nutrient saturation, acupuncture and herbs, and then being aware of when each organ was energised so as not to do the things that further deplete chi and blood. This way he could recapture his excitement for business without such a high physical and emotional cost.

HEART DISEASE

A lot of people pay too high a price for their success, losing not only joy but also their lives. Heart disease is a leading cause of death in many countries. In western medicine it is attributed to an inadequacy of the heart and blood vessels, and stress, diet and lifestyle are seen as major contributors. In traditional Chinese medicine, heart disease is a symptom and chest pain and heart failure have many causes. The basic one is the obstruction of the circulation of a person's chi and blood. Yes, stress, diet and lifestyle do contribute to this, but if you follow the Perfect Day Plan instructions it won't happen.

In traditional Chinese medicine, heart disease is a symptom and chest pain and heart failure have many causes. The basic one is the obstruction of the circulation of a person's chi and blood.

PURPOSE 101

I had another client, Paul, around the same age as Tony. Paul didn't have the same material success, but felt equally lost and unhappy. He was a compulsive eater, dangerously obese and on heart medication. The only thing he liked about his life was his family. He had spent thirty years in a job he hated, focusing purely on buying a house, paying the bills and getting his kids through school. Now his kids were leaving home and his wife was retraining to be an interior designer, something she had always wanted to do. He felt his life had no purpose so therefore it had no meaning. He just wanted to go fishing.

Fishing or shopping, or whatever does it for you, might give you a temporary sense of purpose but we need something deeper than that. This 'something' is not necessarily going to come from career or achievements. We are not all meant to be missionaries, famous authors, great athletes or spiritual leaders. Purpose is something we *feel*. It comes out of our organs. Kids don't sit around wondering who they are or what their purpose is in life. They live each day to the fullest with lots of playfulness and joy. If your life feels purposeless, step one is to get aboard the chi cycle and try and get organs like a child again. Change your lifestyle and nurture your blood and chi and it will happen. Here's how easy it is to start: get a phone book, turn to the traditional Chinese medicine pages and find somewhere to get Chinese raw herbs and acupuncture. Most cities have a Chinatown—

this means there are practitioners of Chinese medicine at hand. If you don't feel you are on the same page with the practitioner you find, try another one until you have what you need in place.

If you follow the Perfect Day Plan, each day your organs are going to be a bit happier and your heart is going to feel protected and so it will relax. Your worldview will change. You will start waking up for yourself, excited about the day ahead. Your life will feel joyous, meaningful and purposeful.

THE HEART AND THE MID-LIFE CRISIS

The wives of my mid-life crisis clients often say their husbands or partners are cut off from their feelings. This isn't so. The mid-life crisis is fuelled by feelings. It is loss, confusion, nostalgia and emptiness that drives you to fast cars or any other number of activities associated with excitement or feelings you think give you purpose.

But it's the *underlying* condition that needs to be treated. This underlying condition comes from the reverse cycle lifestyle. If you haven't been nurturing your energy or building your blood, your organs have been slowly running

If you haven't been nurturing your energy or building your blood, your organs have been slowly running out of fuel. By the time you hit middle age, the symptoms of this are so obvious you can no longer ignore them.

out of fuel. By the time you hit middle age, the symptoms of this are so obvious you can no longer ignore them. Not understanding this, you try and change the way you feel through cars or shopping or drugs, but the real solution is internal.

The Early Mid-life Crisis

I hit my mid-life crisis in my twenties. I was a heavy drug-user and as the ongoing drug use systematically depleted my chi and blood, my heart was empty, there was no joy in my life and everything was so meaningless I was suicidally depressed. I see plenty of young people who have been living the reverse cycle lifestyle and also end up in the same place.

When you reach this stage of organ depletion, you feel nothing but pain. My advice is, whether you're battling obesity, addiction, depression, psychosis or heart disease, just start doing as many chi-cycle friendly things as possible. Life will improve.

SELF-NEGLECT

Neglecting our chi and blood means neglecting our heart and soul. We will end up feeling not only depressed and purposeless, but rejected, abandoned and unloved. It is all too easy to project this onto others and blame our partners, parents or friends, but it is not their fault. Once you are starting to feel 'ripped-off' in life, it is a sign you are neglecting your chi and your blood.

Once you are starting to feel 'ripped-off' in life, it is a sign you are neglecting your chi and your blood.

It is a common belief that happiness is a result of how we see things and how we think, that it is a choice we can make. In traditional Chinese medicine, you cannot just choose to be happy. If you feel neglected, depressed and purposeless, you can read every success book ever written and it will make no difference. What will make a difference is getting the physical infrastructure for happiness in place—healthy organs, healthy chi and blood.

THE INNER SANCTUM

Our heart must be protected at all costs because it is the inner sanctum where all our mental and physical functions are conceived and coordinated. The brain is more like a processing centre—it is the heart that runs everything. The heart is also the seat of the mind. If you let your chi and blood become depleted your heart feels vulnerable and, as we will see in the 7 to 9 pm pericardium chapter, the outcome can be panic disorders.

In traditional Chinese medicine our heart also holds our memories, which is why we hear stories of heart transplant

Our heart holds our memories, which is why we hear stories of heart transplant recipients suddenly acquiring new skills or memories.

recipients suddenly acquiring new skills or memories. A heart depleted of chi and blood also contributes to poor memory. If you are starting to forget things, don't write reminder lists: build your blood and chi.

THE PERFECT WEDDING DAY

One of my favourite workshop questions about the Perfect Day Plan was from a woman asking the best time of day to get married. It is definitely heart time when 'love' is the word and we can be consciously in touch with our souls. My recommendations for the perfect wedding day would begin the night before. First, guys, don't get drunk on your bucks' night, wake up naked chained to a lamp post then stumble through the wedding day hung-over and dazed. This is not a good way to start a new journey with someone. It can come back to you years later.

Change is always associated with fear. When you get drunk at a hen's party or bucks' night you draw upon the communal strength of your friends to temporarily overcome your fear or doubt. A better way is to transform your fear into action. I'd go to bed early the night before the wedding and get up early on the day and use exercise to resolve any lingering fears you might have. Visualise going on an exciting lifelong adventure with someone you love deeply.

Then at stomach time between 7 and 9 am have a full-hearted wholesome breakfast by yourself. Take 45 minutes to 'arrive'. While you do this, see yourself as a married person and feel good about it. The stomach will ground this idea and make it real. By nine in the morning as you hit spleen time, you will feel centred and know who you are and that you can go for it. In spleen time bring on the action, all the friends and the relatives and their dramas. Get dressed, get to the venue. Start the ceremony at 11 am when your chi moves to your heart and you have access to your soul. It is communion time between you and your spouse. Say the things that are closest to your heart and let the fire element spread them.

LOVE YOURSELF

At heart time 'love' is the word and loving yourself is the action. Living in accordance with the chi cycle is my definition of loving yourself.

At heart time 'love' is the word and loving yourself is the action.

If you do this your blood will be healthy, your chi will be strong and you will have a passion for life and your heart will inspire you to spread the love.

Chapter 5
Slow Down a Little
1 pm to 3 pm

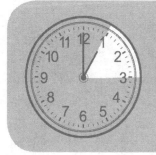

BODY PART – SMALL INTES-
TINE
KEY THOUGHT – SLOW
TIME TO . . .
Have lunch, go slow, ride the
wave

YIN TIME

Between 1 and 3 pm our chi moves from our heart to our
small intestine. The major cyclical shift from a yang into a yin
phase is now seriously kicking in. This transition has a similar
quality to a tidal shift in the ocean; it launches a big energy
change in the day. Understanding this shift and changing our
thoughts and actions from now on is really important.

We should do all our hard work in the yang period of the day. It is as if we are on the upward climb of a giant roller-coaster and now, as our chi moves from our heart to our small intestine, we tip over the peak and it is time to go on the ride.

MEETING THE EDITOR

Our small intestine is paired with our heart, and it too plays a role in 'editing' how we present to the world. Physically, it is responsible for separating the pure and impure and sending the latter to the large intestine for excretion.

Of this organ pairing, the heart is like the good-looking sibling who gets all the attention. Heart imagery adorns everything from greeting cards to bed linen. I recently saw a TV commercial featuring people going about their daily business carrying big fluffy red hearts. The message was that if we saw what we were doing to our hearts by eating badly we would all be much more careful. I really liked the idea (even though the commercial was for margarine rather than the chi cycle).

We need to think about all our organs in this way—even the less glamorous ones such as our small intestine. The commercial wouldn't work as well with people lugging around metres of furry intestines, but the properties of the small intestine are as equally wonderful

If we want to develop spiritually it is crucially important to have a clear mind and make wise decisions.

as the heart's. If we want to develop spiritually it is crucially important to have a clear mind and make wise decisions. The small intestine gives us this mental clarity and wisdom.

EAT LUNCH

Small intestine time is great because you don't have to do anything except eat and relax. The most important thing to do in this two-hour period is have a delicious, nurturing lunch—the biggest meal of the day. To do the right thing by our small intestine, lunch has to be warm and celebratory. I'm not talking about sandwiches here!

Ban the Sandwich

If I was in charge of everything I would ban sandwiches for lunch. Every day in my clinic I treat a stream of stressed-out, angry, anxious, hyper-tense people who are slowly falling apart and don't know why.

They sit there and describe lives totally out of rhythm with the chi cycle. When we get to the part about what they eat, they casually remark that they skip breakfast but then make up for this by having a 'really healthy lunch'. When I ask what this is, the answer is always 'a salad sandwich'. If a rabbit was sitting there telling me that was a good lunch I would agree, because rabbits don't have to do anything.

Though many of us might like to take up this rabbit lifestyle, we can't. We are self-aware. We have responsibilities. We are here to undertake challenges and work with our soul and our destiny. We need to nourish our blood, chi and organs to achieve this. Sandwiches do not do this.

> We need to nourish our blood, chi and organs. Sandwiches do not do this.

Nourishment comes from warm meals containing protein, rice and vegetables. It comes from eating them in heart-warming company, in a nurturing environment. Scoffing sandwiches at your desk between phone calls and appointments, or while rushing around trying to catch up on chores or deal with family is not nourishment. At lunch you have to sit back and eat. If you are with people, talk about joyful things. If you race around or talk about stressful things while you eat it interrupts the processes of refinement in the small intestine. It contributes to time-deprivation, heart disease and, I believe, cancer.

> If you race around or talk about stressful things while you eat it contributes to time-deprivation, heart disease and, I believe, cancer.

The Mediterranean Diet

Lately we have seen a lot of interest in the Mediterranean diet because it has been linked with a lower risk of heart disease and cancer. Various companies try and recapture the essence of this diet, which is high in antioxidants, in tablets or tonics but that is only part of the picture. In Mediterranean cultures they *love* food and they eat lunch joyously with friends or family. You might be able to bottle antioxidants, but you can't bottle this emotion. Even my comparatively glum German kinfolk understand the importance of a warm family lunch.

The problem is most of us now live deep in sandwich territory. Kids are routinely sent off to school with a white-bread sandwich and a couple of biscuits or a piece of fruit for lunch. I don't know how they survive. It is the 'sandwich cultures' that have the high levels of obesity, depression and drug abuse. Perhaps there is a connection. We have to be practical of course. Most of us can't go home for a family lunch and not all of us would want to even if we could, myself included (being with your family is not necessarily joyful or relaxing). So, we have to adapt the concept to suit us.

I had one client, Cynthia, a young, successful and attractive professional, who did this well. Cynthia had the classic high-achiever lifestyle. She worked long hours to stay at the top of her field and had no concept that food was a necessary part of life. Because she had a yang constitution she could get through until the afternoon without eating anything. She routinely skipped breakfast, lived on sandwiches and stress and slowly depleted her organs. She ended up depressed and medicated. Antidepressants made her feel much worse, so she decided to change everything about the way she lived. She embraced the chi cycle and took home-cooked meals to work for lunch. On her lunch break she gathered a couple of work friends together and made them sit down somewhere nice to eat and talk about non-work-related things.

Slowing and Flowing Down

We need to be out of the work environment and not talk about work while we eat lunch, because we want to create the same downward flow of energy we did at breakfast. This downward flow of energy allows absorption of nutrients and contributes to building strong blood and chi which, as we know now, is a critical component of health, happiness and success.

I see a lot of people these days whose energy flow is predominantly upward. As a result they often have a knotted stomach or bloating as soon as they eat, or they can't face a substantial meal and tend to nibble on snacks while on the go. If we want to reduce health issues such as cancer and heart disease, we need to start loving and respecting lunchtime as well as our organs. After lunch the universal forces are calling on us to slow down—the great yin phase of the Perfect Day Plan is underway, and we ignore it at our peril.

SIESTA

The ultimate slow-down is a siesta and between 1 and 3 pm is the ideal time for one. This, of course, is the other aspect of the Mediterranean culture that can't be bottled. In those countries people sit back and relax after a good meal, or even have a nap. They don't rush. Siesta is still respected in many Asian countries as well. I don't think we will be seeing siestas introduced into our time-deprived yang work culture any time in the near future. What we can do, though, is bear the concept of slowness in mind and act accordingly. Try and sit for 10 to 15 minutes after eating lunch. If you read this and immediately think 'I can't do that' you are already on the path to a time/yang pathology and need to re-evaluate how you are living.

TAKE THE BACK SEAT

During small intestine time we have to take the back seat and let the universe do the driving for a while. At work this is the best time to slack off and gossip around the water cooler. Try not to do this in the morning because it wastes the morning's potential productivity. If you have to keep working at small intestine time, do the least taxing things of the day. Don't schedule important meetings, make the big decisions or confront anyone, and don't do anything highly stressful. Don't work gung-ho like you did at spleen time either.

The great sage Lao Tzu said: 'Do your work, then step back. The only path to serenity.' If we don't 'step back', either by allowing ourselves to 'arrive' at breakfast time or sit back for lunch, we are not following the path of yin and yang, we are trying to control yin and yang. This is impossible and it is not healthy.

If we refuse to get in the back seat and insist on trying to stay behind the wheel the entire time, the phrase 'hanging on for grim death' takes on a new meaning. We gradually lose the ability to ever stop and it contributes to the development of what I call an 'additional drive'. Cancer is an example of this and no one wants to go down that path.

Success and the Small Intestine

We are supposed to be doing things in life and going for our goals and seeking success, but in a civilised manner! This means charging ahead sometimes and sitting back at other times. Being able to *not do* things is as important as being able to do things. Living in accord with the chi cycle and the natural forces means respecting the times for not doing things.

> Being able to *not do* things is as important as being able to do things.

If you are a real doer, someone dominated by the drive of a strong yang energy, sitting back is very difficult. Your nature is going to drive you forward. When that nature meets the excitement and urgency of deadlines, goals and the challenges that are part of business, it's a terrific high-energy success combination. But if you keep moving on relentlessly your nature can turn against you and eventually you pay for success with your health, relationship or business. Real success in business and life comes from mastering the art of living.

The forces of yin and yang are always either working for you or against you. There is no neutral position. If you do not have enough time to stop and sit back for lunch or at any other time because you think things will run out of control, what has actually run out of control is your yang. The solution is to build yin to balance this. This allows the periods of hard work to be much more effective and you end up gaining back time for yourself. Following the Perfect Day Plan and living in accord with the chi cycle creates results that working harder never will.

Handover Mode

If you make the time for breakfast and to sit after lunch, you will find you have more time for everything else. So work towards taking 30 minutes for lunch and between 1 and 3 pm switch your mindset to 'handover' mode. The process is similar to a writer handing their manuscript over to an editor. A good book is a team effort and a perfect day also requires teamwork between us, our organs and the natural forces. If we work hard all morning with the backing of the natural forces, we will be so productive that we will be able to hand over some responsibility at small intestine time. This means we get a bit of relief and we can detach from everything, and it is this detachment that allows for mental clarity. That in turn makes us wise.

Sitting Tight

Handing over makes us healthy too. The Perfect Day Plan is designed to keep chi flowing smoothly. If we can't hand over or sit back in small intestine time our chi can't flow on freely to the next organ, which can result in heat and blood stagnation, the road to heart disease. You can actually feel this blockage in the heart and the small intestine meridians which radiate down the left arm. When energy can't flow it leads to rigidity of the mind and change of any sort, whether it is sitting down for lunch, delegating more responsibility to your staff or being nicer to your spouse, will then be out of the question.

Rigidity means we stick to our old lifestyle, then we develop more symptoms like blood pressure, mood swings, depression, digestive disorders and so on.

Medications mask these symptoms and allow us to keep going in the reverse cycle lifestyle. This is not sustainable. It is estimated that 60 per cent of the US population is on medication. When you add the 40 per cent estimated to be using recreational drugs, and the fact that we now have four- and five-year-olds on heavy duty attention deficit disorder drugs or even anti-psychotics, it is pretty evident that the reverse cycle is not the way to live. We need to start thinking about and practising another way of living. The chi cycle and flowing along with the forces of yin and yang is the only way.

CHILL

In each 24-hour cycle, there are times when we have to sit back, be in our bodies and feel the pull of the earth. We don't have to dress in cheesecloth or hug a tree to do this. It doesn't matter whether we are in an underground car park, an office block or our lounge room. We just need to be aware of where our chi or energy is and what we should be doing at that time, and things will change.

Being able to sit back during lunch and at other times during the chi cycle when required, regardless of how intense the situation around you is, means food goes down, nutrients are absorbed,

Learn to chill out at small intestine time; let yourself receive mental clarity and wisdom.

energy flows and you are more likely to be receiving energy from the universe. So learn to chill out at small intestine time; let yourself receive mental clarity and its offshoot of wisdom, and look forward to another great two hours during bladder time!

Chapter 6
Powering Forward
3 pm to 5 pm

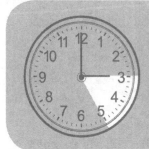

BODY PART – BLADDER
KEY THOUGHT – SUPPORT
TIME TO . . .
Put cruise control on, go with the flow, feel the power

ALLIANCE

At 3 pm our chi moves from our small intestine to our bladder and we shift from the fire element to the water element. By now, following the Perfect Day Plan, we would have had a nice warm breakfast somewhere between 7 and 9 am. Then we worked really hard between 9 and 11 am, got in touch with our soul between 11 am and 1 pm, had a warm, joyous, nutritious lunch and allowed ourselves to sit back somewhere between 1 pm and 3 pm in small intestine time. As a result, all our organs are working together to deliver their magic. All that good food, hard work and positive thinking has been offered to our heart and converted into such healthy blood any vampire would give their right arm for it.

Our heart pulses with life energy and we are happy people who radiate joy and love. We have accepted the gifts of each two-hour block: emotional balance, self-development, soul purpose, wisdom and clarity of mind. This is already a pretty nice gift pack, but it keeps getting better. The water element is the basis of all physical life and between 3 and 5 pm we should sense a rising of hope and feel as if we are getting a new lease on life.

SENDING IN THE TROOPS

The bladder channel, the longest meridian in the body, is packed with acupuncture points. It is connected with 'backbone', and in bladder time we can feel the support of the universal energy.

Bladder time is when we get a taste of the rewards of living in harmony with the forces of yin and yang. The bladder channel, the longest meridian in the body, is packed with acupuncture points that offer direct access to all the organs. It is connected with 'backbone', and in bladder time we can feel the support of the universal energy. It is like that scene in movies where the small group of warriors have been valiantly battling against a much bigger force. Just as they think they can't go on, a huge army appears on the horizon to help out and they get carried to victory. But we can only feel this if we are tapped into the chi cycle.

In traditional Chinese medicine perfection is a vision, not a reality. It is more likely that we got up late and staggered out of bed towards a caffeine hit. We started off the day feeling like crap and carrying all our baggage with us. Then we added to it by rushing, scoffing down cold cereal and tearing off to work or into our tasks for the day. We never 'arrived' and this means it is going to be a hopeless race to catch up all day. By 10 am we feel so tired we need more caffeine and a sugar hit to keep moving. We haven't got the energy to work hard during spleen time, so we slack off and waste time, then fall behind and have to work hard, not smart, through heart time. We feel no connection to our soul or destiny; we use up more of our chi reserves, then we commit the sin of having a sandwich at small intestine time and keep pushing on.

THREE-THIRTY-ITIS

As a result of our less-than-perfect reality 3 to 5 pm becomes one of the worst times of the day. When we get to three-thirty, instead of feeling our universal support we

> When we get to three-thirty, instead of feeling support we feel alone, exhausted and weak. We have to drag ourselves through these two hours.

feel alone, exhausted and weak. We have to drag ourselves through these two hours. This is the time when most accidents happen due to negligence and poor decision-making. In Japan they have special bars where people can invigorate themselves at three-thirty with oxygen or a nutrient drip. In the west people go for chocolate, biscuits or cake and more caffeine to get them through the rest of the afternoon. But three-thirty-itis is the symptom of depleted blood and chi, and sugar and stimulants will only make this worse.

The good news is that this can be reversed at any time, simply by getting in tune with the chi cycle. Sticking to the Perfect Day Plan will gradually change everything because each action which is in harmony with the cycle makes the next stage more likely to be in harmony and so on. It starts a movement of ever-increasing energy and vitality.

CRUISE CONTROL

By 3 pm we should have done all the pushing for the day. The yin phase that picked up momentum in small intestine time is continuing to build and we should go along with this by using the impetus of our actions so far to carry us forward. In the previous two hours between 1 and 3 pm, we sat in the back seat and let the universe do the driving. Now, in bladder time, we get behind the wheel again but put on the cruise control.

Having cruise control on doesn't mean heading for the couch and TV (that comes later).

We continue working, but do the easier tasks of the day. Between 3 and 5 pm our work should be enjoyable, not hard. We don't

Between 3 and 5 pm our work should be enjoyable, not hard.

want to exploit our own energy stores at this time of the day. The morning should have been so productive that we can now tackle the more routine jobs that don't require the same level of energy and creative input, but still need to be done. Unimportant meetings, routine correspondence, paperwork, processing, accounts and other mundane tasks are perfect for bladder time.

If you are not at work, between 3 and 5 pm is the best time of the chi cycle to do the grocery shopping. Put your headphones on and wander through the aisles semi-automatically. You are still doing something that has to be done but not in an urgent manner.

However, 3 to 5 pm is another time of day where we may face the inability to hand over anything. I have many clients who can't stop pushing because they are worried that if they do, everything will collapse. This exaggerated sense of responsibility arises partially because they have never experienced the backup that comes from the universal energy,

We have ended up in the crazy situation where many people think slowing down or sitting back is a sign of weakness or a waste of time.

but also because they don't have the skills or the desire to let go. We have actually ended up in the crazy situation where many people think slowing down or sitting back is a sign of weakness or a waste of time.

This only happens because we are out of touch with the natural rhythms and forces of yin and yang. If you are one of these people, try and keep the idea of cruise control in mind between 3 and 5 pm. Aim to do things in a more relaxed way until five o'clock, when your chi moves to your kidneys and the party starts.

LEARNING TO NOT DO

In the previous chapter we saw that 'not doing' is as important as 'doing'. A key to our health and happiness, and to feeling supported in the afternoon at bladder time, is learning to sit back at small intestine time. In the Perfect Day Plan, up until 1 pm all our yang activities of working, achieving and so on have been developing chi. But by three each afternoon all the effort and production of the previous hours are supposed to have been transformed into a yin quality to balance the yang. Sitting back and going slow after lunch starts this off.

If we keep on working really hard against the flow of the natural forces we keep building our yang, which can create insomnia, emotional instability, frustration, anger and other uncomfortable states. If we follow the chi cycle it will take us back to the way life should be and during bladder time we will have a powerful reminder of how good it feels to be a child of the universe.

Chapter 7
Drift a Little

5 pm to 7 pm

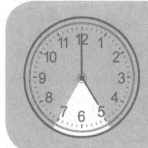

BODY PART – KIDNEYS
KEY THOUGHT – SWITCH OFF
TIME TO . . .
Acknowledge strength and skills,
have sex, share a laugh

PARTY ON!

By 5 pm each day our chi moves to our kidneys and it is party time! For the next two hours we are up for drinking, laughing, bragging, sex and, um, maybe also some reflection on the day. These two hours are also all about yin and yang because in traditional Chinese medicine our kidneys are said to be the 'mother of yin and yang'. If we have managed to live in harmony with the cycle through the day, we have also been making yin and yang work for us and this is a great secret of success. If we can keep our next actions in flow with the natural forces as well, when our chi enters our kidneys it is just going to get better and better.

Around 5 pm the workday is finishing and most people are preparing to go home. On a spiritual level we are also starting the process of 'returning home'. So the most important thing to do between 5 and 7 pm is consciously switch over from all the yang activities of the day to a yin mode, so that this process can take place.

HYDRO POWER

We are still in the water element at kidney time. Water is the most powerful life-giving element in the physical world and our kidneys are the most powerful organ in our body. So this is a really awesome time of the day. It is a time of power. But kidney time should be spent reflecting on that power, not exploiting it. We reflect on it by acknowledging our strengths and skills.

> This is a really awesome time of the day. Kidney time should be spent reflecting on that power, not exploiting it, by acknowledging our strengths and skills.

If you use your kidney-time power to keep on working you create excess mental energy, which leads to insomnia. If we can't sleep, we can't get up early enough to get a perfect day underway and we will be chasing something that eludes us for the rest of the day. By the next 5 pm kidney time we are too far behind to stop; we have no hope of switching off and on it goes. This lifestyle wastes energy. It traps you in the rat race and leads to depression, defeat, medication and negativity.

ACCESS TO THE ENGINE ROOM

At kidney time we must switch off. Between 5 and 7 pm it is as if the door to the powerhouse, to your internal engine room, is open. So you need to get in there before it shuts and throw your inner power switch to 'off'. This is the only time of day when you have this access.

Switching off determines not only your ability to sleep, but also the quality of your sleep. Sleep is the ultimate yin activity. As we will see, really important things happen while you are asleep which are essential to your physical, spiritual and emotional health.

Throwing the Switch

So how do you throw the switch at kidney time? One option is go to the pub, have a couple of drinks with your friends, brag about your achievements or joke about the dramas of the day. When you are in the thick of those problems, you are generally unable to laugh. But if at kidney time you find the funny side and share it with friends, you are actually acknowledging your strengths and skills but also, because you can laugh at stressful events, embracing an opposite state. This is exactly what you are supposed to be doing at kidney time. It's a great example of switching from yang to yin. It matches the intelligence of the kidneys.

Even though 5 to 7 pm is a powerful time of day, you don't want to still be going hard at kidney time. If you like that feeling, though, you can use sex to switch off. Between 5 and 7 pm is the best time of the whole 24 hours for sex, because our chi is in the kidneys—the organ associated with sexual energy. Sex at this time also fits in with what we are supposed to be doing because it is another, perhaps more loving way of 'embracing the opposite', of switching from yang to yin.

> Between 5 and 7 pm is the best time of the whole 24 hours for sex, because our chi is in the kidneys—the organ associated with sexual energy.

NOT TONIGHT DEAR, I'VE GOT A HEADACHE

Many people are not into sex any more, for a variety of reasons. One of the most basic is to do with your organs, chi and blood. If they are healthy and your kidney chi is strong, you will naturally have a balanced appetite for sex. Weak or deficient blood is usually the cause of sexual disinterest in women and weak kidneys the cause for sexual disinterest in men.

> Weak or deficient blood is usually the cause of sexual disinterest in women and weak kidneys the cause for sexual disinterest in men.

In my work I often treat clients who say they are so sexually incompatible with their partner, they are thinking of splitting up. By incompatible they mean one partner wants sex and the other doesn't. They talk about going to get relationship counselling, but blood, chi, kidney and other deficiencies are often the real problems. Counselling won't resolve this, and neither will Viagra or any other such drugs. Before seeing a counsellor, try building your blood and kidney chi by taking Chinese raw herbs and supplements and following the Perfect Day Plan. You'll be amazed how much your sex drive improves.

Obviously you can't have sex every afternoon to switch off and you wouldn't want to anyway as this is not healthy—unless you are young. Young men (15–25 years old) naturally recuperate the energy released in ejaculation within 12 to 24 hours. In adults (30–50 years old) this can take between three and seven days. You can't go to the pub and drink every afternoon either. Another option is to meet friends and exchange your experiences of the day. Taking the kids to the park or having a relaxing massage is another good way to switch from yang to yin. If you are by yourself at this time of day, find somewhere peaceful to sit and remind yourself that you are shifting from doing to non-doing, from goal setting to 'no setting'. Call up the stressors and discomforts of your day and visualise embracing them. The more practice you get at this, the easier it becomes.

THE THREE-THIRTY-ITIS HANGOVER

In the previous chapter we looked at three-thirty-itis, a classic symptom arising from not understanding the need for balancing yin and yang in life and from getting caught up in deadlines, thinking everything is urgent and having no time for sitting back. Exhausted, depleted and lethargic, we try and invigorate ourselves with chocolate bars, energy drinks or double-shot coffees. Unfortunately, after a while the lethargy comes back worse than before as your yin is now even less capable of balancing a very toxic yang.

> By kidney time at 5 pm, instead of feeling power you feel the three-thirty-itis hangover hitting. Everything moves far too slowly, everyone annoys you.

As a result, by kidney time at 5 pm, instead of feeling power you feel the three-thirty-itis hangover hitting. You become reactive, unpredictable and prone to road rage or other uncontrollable outbursts. Everything moves far too slowly, everyone annoys you. By the time you get home, you've had it. Everyone there annoys you too so you actively look for confrontation, or you just want to get drunk or turn to dope or prescribed pills to control your irritability, depression or self-doubt and forget about the day.

Drink and Drugs and Yin and Yang

Getting drunk (which is very different from having a couple of drinks with friends to relax) in an attempt to forget about the day can make switching off even harder. Alcohol can make your yang rise, increase anger and get you all heated up. By bedtime you can't bring your yang down. The doors to the engine room are locked tight, your opportunity to throw the switch is gone and you will be unable to sleep.

By 7 pm you need to have consciously handed over the quarrels and stresses of the day to the motherly embrace of your kidneys. Otherwise you will be taking the stresses to bed. Once your problem boss, nasty clients, toxic relatives and grudges jump in to bed with you, no one is going to get any sleep. Then you can't get up in the morning, can't face breakfast, and it kicks off another reverse cycle day.

By 7 pm you need to have consciously handed over the quarrels and stresses of the day to the motherly embrace of your kidneys. Otherwise you will be taking the stresses to bed.

Peace, Man

Between 5 and 7 pm is the time to make peace with your challenges, trials and discomforts. Lay them to rest for the next ten or twelve hours. Be accepting of the views of others. Avoid confrontational situations as this prevents you embracing the opposite and prevents the kidneys from doing their job of switching from yang to yin.

FORGING ON

If you have to keep working between 5 and 7 pm, try not to be overwhelmed by the demands on you. Keep reminding yourself that this is kidney time, a time when everything is fine, everything is good, everything is perfect. Even if you can only tell yourself this for 5 minutes at 6.50 pm it will still have an effect. Devote a few minutes to it here and there and it will allow you to slowly begin to harmonise your actions with kidney time. Your stress levels will drop and your sleep will improve. The more skills you apply at kidney time, the more in control of your life you will be.

GYM JUNKIES

A lot of people go to the gym between 5 and 7 pm, forcing themselves through a gruelling work-out, thinking they are burning off all the stress and frustration of the day. This is not switching off, unless of course for you running hard on the treadmill is as good as having a few drinks with close friends or having terrific sex. If you do want to go to the gym during kidney time, put on your exercise gear but take a bottle of wine and spend your time there wandering around, wineglass in hand, chatting to everyone about what you did that day.

Exercising is not a method for 'switching off' in the way your kidneys need. And doing it between 5 and 7 pm is not effective in terms of physical fitness or weight loss. It requires an active metabolism for a minimum of ten hours following the exercise for it to contribute to weight loss, but after working out in the evening you are going home to relax. Your metabolism

> Exercising is not a method for 'switching off' in the way your kidneys need. And doing it between 5 and 7 pm is not effective in terms of physical fitness or weight loss.

immediately slows down. As we will see, exercise belongs in the early morning.

Our kidney time switching-off activities need to be effective because happiness does not come from yang followed by yang, it comes from balancing yin and yang and accepting that we will never finish all our tasks. If we do the right things at kidney time it helps lay the foundation for peace in our lives, as our chi moves to our pericardium, the delicate membrane that surrounds our heart.

Chapter 8
Get Creative
7 pm to 9 pm

BODY PART – PERICARDIUM
KEY THOUGHT – PROTECT
TIME TO ...
Come home, be yourself, be creative, have dinner

BE SAFE

By seven each evening our chi moves to our pericardium, the membrane that surrounds our heart. In traditional Chinese medicine the pericardium's job is to protect our heart, the seat of our mind and soul. The psychological and emotional associations of the pericardium are protection and safety; so what we need to do between 7 and 9 pm, to help our pericardium help our heart, is allow ourselves to feel 'at home'.

In acupuncture the pericardium channel is one of the most important for treating stress. We can activate stress relief ourselves by what we do in the next two hours. So, somewhere in pericardium time, relax by yourself or with family, put your feet up and simply be yourself. It is not about switching off—we did that somewhere in the previous two hours of kidney time—it is about allowing our chi to flow smoothly in the pericardium channel so it can let the tension of the day melt away.

> In pericardium time, relax by yourself or with family, put your feet up and simply be yourself.

We are back in the fire element at pericardium time. It is the only element that appears twice in the 24-hour cycle. I like to think of that fire as warming up our heart and soul.

NEGLECTING OUR DUTIES

If you have lived in accordance with the Perfect Day Plan so far, 7 to 9 pm is a lovely time because you will be feeling stress-free, cosy and safe in yourself. However, if you have been working late, skipping meals and not switching off, you get home but can't relax then you can't sleep, lie in bed scratching at your skin and can't get up the next day, and stress builds and builds. This makes it hard to feel safe, and leaves your heart vulnerable. This is why we have such a big problem these days with heart disease and panic and anxiety disorders.

THE HIT PARADE

The job of our organs is to protect the heart. They pay the price for our reverse cycle actions. Our liver is the first to cop it. As its energy stagnates we start feeling irritable and frustrated and have flare-ups of unreasonable anger. Then our spleen follows and we lose our appetite for good food and start craving sweets. We worry obsessively about trivial things, we can't concentrate and feel permanently fatigued. The kidneys go next and we lose power over our lives, lack sex drive or become over-sexed. We develop lower back pain and frequent urination. Our lungs hold out as long as possible but, as each organ is depleted of chi, the next organ has to work even harder and crashes more quickly. When our lung energy declines immunity breaks down, so we get sick all the time. We are always exhausted and short of breath at the slightest exertion. We live in the past and fear the future.

If you have any of these symptoms and continue your life-style unchanged or medicate your discomfort away, eventually your organs will be overloaded and can't protect your heart. Now it is up to the pericardium, the last gatekeeper before the heart. Your pericardium is like a super-efficient personal

The pericardium is like an envelope, and it is as if each night it collects up all the bad things we have said and done, thought and eaten and stores them so the heart doesn't need to stress about any of it.

assistant who really worries about the boss and does everything they can to protect them. The pericardium is a double-skinned membrane, like an envelope, and it is as if each night it collects up all the bad things we have said and done, thought and eaten and stores them so the heart doesn't need to stress about any of it.

Our job is to follow the Perfect Day Plan as it enables us to live in a way that empties out that envelope each day so our organs can start to recover. If we don't the pericardium storage gets so full, it starts squeezing the heart. The heart suddenly realises everything is out of control. It had no idea. It freaks out. It races madly and we get palpitations.

Under siege

When the pericardium's storage is full the heart feels besieged so we don't feel safe. The outcome can be anxiety and panic attacks. I have been seeing a lot of clients lately who are suddenly experiencing this in their late forties and early fifties. They often think they are having a heart attack. Panic attacks are evidence that your life is so off-course physically and/or spiritually that your organs are not functioning as they should and it is time for a serious change.

In traditional Chinese medicine it is said we see the world through our organs. Panic attacks are a fantastic example of the truth of this. Once our organs reach a certain point of depletion and we feel unsafe, normal things start looking dangerous. Before I followed the full chi-cycle life, I had severe panic attacks for several months. One of the things that freaked me out the most were underground car parks—I simply couldn't go into them.

> Once our organs reach a certain point of depletion and we feel unsafe, normal things start looking dangerous.

Panic Merchants

If an innocent car park or streets that you know like the back of your hand suddenly seem strange or threatening, your inner world needs urgent attention. Your organs and heart are not feeling as safe as they should be. But often we don't get this message and instead of changing things we start panicking about the panic attacks.

At this point most people head off to a doctor and start taking medication. After the day I managed to park my car underground but was then unable to retrieve it, I did the same. It was a Z3 convertible and I loved that car, so I knew something had to change. Luckily, the doctor I saw also suffered from panic attacks and told me medication wouldn't help. In her opinion it was all psychological and the solution was to re-program my mind.

This might work for some people, but with my clients I take the opportunity to address the panic attacks physically as well. Organ depletion and stress can be reversed by building blood and chi. Eventually the heart feels safe and the external world changes accordingly. When your blood and organs are nice and healthy the world looks and feels totally different—a warm, loving place you feel at home in.

Inner Insecurity

There are plenty of signs for us prior to panic attacks developing. Feelings of emotional insecurity are an early indicator but, because most people don't know where these feelings come from or the connection between their organs and their emotions, the first thing they do is look outwards for the cause. They may blame their partner, believing he or she is not providing them with the love or attention they need, and their behaviour changes subtly to reflect this. As the partner probably has depleted blood or organs as well, in no time you have kicked off a downward relationship spiral.

> The minute you feel negative emotions—whether it is anger, insecurity or paranoia—it is an indication that you are low on chi or blood or nutrients.

Counselling can't help with this, because the real problem is *physical*.

The minute you feel negative emotions—whether it is anger, insecurity or paranoia—it is an indication that you are low on chi or blood or nutrients. To change the situation you have to change the way you are living. Once you are feeling self-hatred, self-doubt or other negative emotions, you can't change this on the spot but need to change the way you live. Meanwhile, look at these emotions as something to work *with*. Keep remembering that the only problem is the way you are treating yourself.

External Security

Another thing many people do when they feel insecure is subconsciously try and balance this uneasy feeling by working on *external* security. Balance is definitely the right idea, but focusing on the external is the wrong way to go about this. Savings in the bank, owning a home or business or getting a promotion won't help your organs. The negative feelings will keep surfacing in different ways until you get to the point where the discomfort is too strong to ignore and you have to make things change. Go for external

Home isn't necessarily a physical home. I know a lot of people who are home in the evening, but they don't *feel* at home. Feeling at home comes from within.

security by all means, but focus on building *inner* security as well.

At pericardium time allow yourself to 'come home' as this helps create inner security. Home isn't necessarily a physical home. I know a lot of people who are home in the evening, but they don't *feel* at home. Feeling at home comes from within. I travel a lot for business and often find myself spending my pericardium time at the airport or in a plane. These are not comforting, warm or nurturing environments by any stretch of the imagination, but I work on establishing the feeling of being at home regardless of where I am.

CREATIVE TIME

Between 7 and 9 pm is a good time to be creative. In fact anywhere between 5 and 9 pm is. Playing music or doing some form of craft or hobby is a terrific way to 'switch off' but also a sure-fire way to make yourself feel at home. Remember that you must be doing this for *yourself*, not for your boss or job. If you are a designer, you can't bring work home and kid yourself that doing it during pericardium time is okay because it is creative.

Pericardium time is perfect for a ceramics class, life drawing or knitting group, or for reading a great book. In the pre-TV days pericardium time was when the family gathered and did traditional crafts. This nurtured the heart and strengthened family bonds, and also allowed people to feel safe and at home. I don't think family crochet sessions will be making a comeback any time soon, and I wouldn't join in if they did. You need to find something that works for you. I always spend 45 minutes in pericardium time playing music. I can be myself and allow my soul to come forward. As this happens the muscles around my heart relax, and all sense of urgency and stress disappears. I feel at one with the moment and my heart responds accordingly. I feel at peace.

GET YOUR GEAR OFF

Because of our work culture a good part of each day is spent not truly being ourselves, so it's really important to be yourself at pericardium time. Between 7 and 9 pm, a physical way to remind yourself of this is to get changed. During the day most of us have to wear work clothes of some sort and act in accord with others' expectations. Getting out of your 'uniform' and into your own clothes, whether that is a tracksuit, casual clothes, cross-dressing or a chicken-suit, helps create the right frame of mind for pericardium time. Before you get your new gear on, though, or after in some cases, remind yourself that anywhere between 5 and 10 pm is still a good time to have sex!

TV TIME

Pericardium time is also the best time in the chi cycle to watch TV. Doing so allows you to relax and let others do the work for you. In my experience, the benefit of TV declines rapidly after an hour or so. I'd limit viewing time as much as possible, and also be selective about what I watch. I rarely see, read or listen to the news. This is the worst thing to do at any time of the day because inevitably it is negative and do we really need to add that to our existing stress? I think not.

EAT DINNER

Between 7 and 9 pm is the best time to have dinner.

Between 7 and 9 pm is the best time to have dinner. Many people eat around six believing it is a healthy thing to do, but if you are following the chi cycle you'll find that eating dinner around seven-thirty works best. Timing your evening meal for seven-thirty still provides enough time for the food to settle before going to bed and will give you sufficient energy to get up enthusiastically in the morning. I usually have a snack around 5 pm such as almonds and apples to keep myself going, then have a simple meal for dinner.

The ideal dinner is a lighter version of lunch.

The ideal dinner is a lighter version of lunch. These days most people skip breakfast, have a sandwich for lunch then focus on a big cooked dinner. This is the reverse of what your organs want. I would put the emphasis on a good warm breakfast and lunch, then don't worry so much about dinner. It can be salads, vegies, rice and protein—if you need it. Most of us are yin deficient and protein builds yin. I add protein powder to my breakfast porridge, I always have a good source of protein for lunch and usually a smaller portion for dinner.

Sandwich Time

For all those sandwich lovers out there, the good news is that pericardium time is also the best time of the chi cycle to have toast or sandwiches. Bread or other wheat products like pasta make you tired—which is why they are a no-no for breakfast or lunch—but at pericardium time being tired is not necessarily a bad thing. I have to say, though, I wouldn't even eat bread then. I think bread is something you can have when you are young, but by the time you get to around forty you want to ditch it and other wheat products from your diet. It really bloats and distorts the body. If you want to see a marked change in your body shape, stop eating bread (and sugar and cheese!).

During pericardium time, universal yin is building and things should be slowing down. This continues until midnight when the yin peaks. The actions of pericardium time, of returning home, of being yourself, of warming your soul by being creative and eating a light meal are all in tune with this yin movement. They are a pre-requisite for sleep and all the amazing spiritual activities that are to follow as our chi moves to our san jiao (see Chapter 9).

Chapter 9
Time to Sleep
9 pm to 11 pm

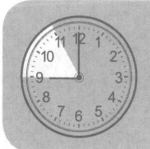

BODY PART – SAN JIAO
KEY THOUGHT – PASSAGE
TIME TO ...
Snuggle up in bed, drift away

THE BEGINNING AND THE END OF CHI

At 9 pm our chi moves to the san jiao. This is a very mysterious organ. It is invisible and there has been much debate as to whether it is an organ or just a function. Either way, in traditional Chinese medicine the san jiao is part of our organ system and it plays a really important role in the chi cycle. It is said to be the beginning and end of chi, probably because the san jiao controls the movement of various types of chi or energy at different times in the 24-hour chi cycle. But we don't need to know the mechanics of that, just as we don't need to know how our TV works. What we do need to know is that the gift of san jiao time is 'passage'. This is that delicious feeling of being snuggled up in bed and feeling yourself drifting away—falling or passing from one plane of existence to another.

GO TO BED

The most important thing to do at san jiao time between 9 and 11 pm is go to bed. And don't take anything with you, except your partner or your teddy bear. Our sleep is so crucial we should think of our bedroom as a temple. I'd make the room look like this sort of place as much as possible too, as a physical reminder of the importance of what happens while we are asleep.

Each night at the door of the temple get in the right frame of mind for what is about to happen. Take off your shoes and hand in your laptop and anything work related or stressful. By now, if you have been following the Perfect Day Plan, you should have already alleviated all your stress during kidney and pericardium times by switching off and letting yourself feel safe and at home. This prepares the ground for the san jiao to do its work and deliver your 'passage'.

Wreckage in Bed

Many people take a book, a cup of tea and some biscuits to bed. Eating in bed is another thing on the banned list! It is right up there with sugar and sandwiches. As we have seen in the previous chapters, to build blood and chi we should be eating at certain times of the day and none of these is bedtime. The san jiao is trying to release toxic chi and arrange your passage to somewhere fantastic. Sitting there putting in sugar and stimulants is not very helpful. It will affect how you sleep and contributes to an internal situation that is going to cost you precious chi. Have tea and biscuits and read books in a comfy armchair at pericardium time, or in bed on your feast day. On the other days, leave off the caffeine or sugar after 4 pm.

While we are on the subject, breakfast in bed is even worse than snacking at night. We are supposed to be up and doing things for a couple of hours before eating, so we can eliminate toxins and fuel up with chi for a new day. The last thing you want to do the minute you open your eyes is start stuffing more toxins down your throat. If you love having breakfast in bed put it on your feast-day list, but somewhere near the bottom!

BAD VIBE, MAN

Everything is chi (or energy), everything accumulates chi. Not all chi is beneficial; some is toxic. Even though you may never have heard of the chi cycle, you know when you walk into a place that has toxic chi because you instinctively get a 'bad vibe' about it. The same happens when you meet certain people. None of us are pure; we all have resistance to things ranging from not wanting to go to work on Monday to driving in traffic. Our resistance creates toxic chi which we then carry around with us. As it accumulates, it affects others.

A bedroom also accumulates chi. Once you become sensitive to this you can feel it. Hotel rooms in particular are overflowing with toxic chi from the various activities that have taken place in them. Before I sleep in a hotel room, I use a chi technique to clear out the old energy.

> In our own bedrooms we want to try and keep the chi as restful as possible.

In our own bedrooms we want to try and keep the chi as restful as possible so we can sleep peacefully. Eating in bed doesn't help with this. I suggest keeping food consumption to the kitchen or stomach room. Do your computer work in your study or spleen room. Read in the lounge, the pericardium room. Sleep and have sex in the temple/bedroom and I think we all know what to do in the 'bowel room'!

BEDTIME

The bed is the altar of the temple and ideally we shouldn't do anything in it except sleep and have sex. A lot of couples start serious relationship discussions once they get to bed. This is also a big no-no. You want to hand in your relationship issues at the bedroom door, as well as all your work-related material. Your organs are not supporting verbal communication or resolution at this time of night. Your emotions are supposed to be settling down, not getting stirred up. Starting these conversations in bed will go nowhere and interfere with your ability to sleep.

Ideally you would talk about tricky relationship issues at spleen time between 9 and 11 am. Another opportunity to talk about your relationship is 5 to 7 pm during kidney time, when we are listening to and embracing an opposite value. These are the times when you have universal support for such discussions, so you will have a better chance of resolution and won't be wasting energy and throwing yourself further off cycle.

Men and Sex

One of the issues that often comes up when people do have bedtime chats is sex. San jiao is a time when people think about sex, either about having it or avoiding it. Many of us instinctively do things that resonate with our organ functions at certain times without knowing it. The energetics of san jiao time are connected with 'letting out chi'. Letting out sperm feels as if it lets out the build-up of the day, which is why many men naturally want to have sex between 9 and 11 pm. If partner-sex is not on the menu, many masturbate then fall asleep. They are using ejaculation as a passage into the sleep state.

Men and women have different needs during san jiao time. Generally speaking, men are influenced more by their kidneys, the organ associated with power. Having sex can create the impression of a release of power. This allows a change of state to yin, which makes falling asleep easier.

Women and Sex

While men are influenced by their kidneys, women's libidos are influenced more by their liver and blood. If they are eating on the run, dieting or eating non-nutritious food, the outcome is blood depletion. This is particularly the case for women who have children and a job, but affects all women. You can feel dizzy, nauseous, emotionally unstable, depressed, empty and exhausted all at the same time. Naturally the last thing you want to do when you get to bed is outlay more effort and energy having sex. Sleep is crucial for women's blood production, health and wellbeing, so you are more likely to want to fall asleep at san jiao time.

AVOIDING BLOOD DEFICIENCY

Having a job and kids is the reality of the 21st century. The answer is not to head to the hills for a tree-change but to have a chi-change. Use the chi cycle to make your lifestyle sustainable. Get on to Chinese raw herbs, protein powder and super-foods a.s.a.p. and you will be able to build up your blood.

Many female clients with blood deficiency tell me they don't take any nutritional supplements because they have a healthy diet. Half of them are vegetarian for starters, so they are automatically in trouble. I don't know why people think vegetarianism automatically means good health. It doesn't. Unless you do the research into foods and protein sources, being vegetarian usually automatically means blood depletion and low energy. Vegetarianism is a great idea for many reasons and something I believe we should aspire to. But the countries that have a primarily vegetarian diet have a culture and cuisine that supports it that was established over centuries. We are a culture that has eaten meat for centuries. You can't just suddenly decide to give it up, eat salad sandwiches and expect to keep functioning.

The only vegetarians I have met who have really healthy blood, strong organs and lots of energy are yang types with naturally high energy levels who also devote hours each day to cooking and combining foods in ways that provide the correct protein intake. We have become a nutrient- and yin-deficient culture. Eating protein is one of the things that provides yin and nutrients. Be vegetarian by all means but be prepared to make the effort to get in tune with the chi cycle and get enough protein from other sources. Not only will your sex drive improve but so will every aspect of your relationship. The two are connected.

> Be vegetarian by all means but be prepared to make the effort to get in tune with the chi cycle and get enough protein from other sources. Not only will your sex drive improve but so will every aspect of your relationship. The two are connected.

Not wanting sex is not purely the outcome of blood depletion; it is also related to emotional imbalances. This means that irrelevant things from the toothpaste tube to the toilet seat will set you off at another person. These all rise out of living the reverse cycle. In fact, all our problems do. After years as a therapist I believe all major problems, local and global, are based on emotional reactivity and a population of individuals that have not resolved themselves. If we follow the Perfect Day Plan we build blood, chi and world peace. This is a great journey to take as a couple because as your health and happiness improves, life will look brighter and brighter every day.

Sex and Drugs

So many women are losing interest in sex that the hunt is on for sexual performance-enhancing drugs for women. Pharmaceutical companies are racing to find the 'female Viagra'. But drugs don't address organ imbalances—they contribute to them. Whereas once the issue for a lot of men was wanting sex every night, now they are struggling with erectile dysfunction or lack of interest in sex. So they turn to drugs to get an erection. These drugs achieve this by forcing blood into the penis. But if you have erectile dysfunction your blood and chi are deficient. Your body needs to conserve what it has. Performance-enhancing drugs divert your blood away from vital functions. This is why heart attacks are often associated with them. If you have an erectile dysfunction it is more than likely going to be related to your chi and blood, and the solution is too.

Sex and the Chi Cycle

If we follow the Perfect Day Plan and build our blood we develop a more balanced sex drive. Generally speaking, for men in normal health and aged from 30 to 45 years old you would be looking at having sex somewhere around three times a week. The ultimate time for it is between 5 and 7 pm (not in the morning or really late at night) as you have the universe and your kidneys backing you up. Too little sex is as bad as too much. Sperm is constantly being produced and refraining from ejaculation for long periods of time is as unhealthy as overdoing it. Not ejaculating for a man is like a woman suppressing a period. Both the production of menstrual blood and sperm are part of a natural cycle.

But ejaculation does chew up a lot of resources. If you are ejaculating daily or several times a day and are not nurturing your chi and your blood, you are heading for erectile dysfunction. Our current yang lifestyle is not helping. It can create 'heat' conditions, which can manifest as an insatiable sex drive. Frequent masturbation can make the condition worse. Having lots of sessions with a sex worker isn't the solution either—a change of lifestyle and sexual technique is!

To get the yin quality to offset that yang, men need to climax after the female. This allows the absorption of yin and then the yang is balanced, otherwise all they are doing is building yang and never feeling satisfied. This increases the urge to have more sex and it becomes a cycle of heat, depletion, yang and sex. The interesting thing about sex and the chi cycle is that the system is actually designed so that men have to make a bit of an effort and do some homework on pleasing their partner because this is ultimately going to benefit them.

Getting aligned with the chi cycle allows you to get in touch with your energy, and gain insight into how yin and yang can work for you. This will impact on your understanding and control of your sex drive. If you then work towards increasing sexual excitement and intensity in your partner before you come it will feel much more satisfying for you both. It will have a positive effect on your health and your relationship as you are much more likely to be a satisfying lover. Also, with a more balanced sex drive, the urge to ejaculate every night decreases and the san jiao can do its job of letting chi out.

> With a more balanced sex drive, the urge to ejaculate every night decreases.

Good Sex, Good Relationship

Many clients who have an unsatisfactory sex life tell me sex isn't important. I disagree—sex does matter. We are all sensual creatures and need each other's touch. In a harmonious relationship both partners have an equal desire for sex. Whether it's once a day, once a week, once a month, once a year or not at all, it doesn't matter, so long as it is mutually agreeable.

If both partners want sex at san jiao time, great, go for it. For many couples this is the only time they get physically close and can have sex. It's a great way to prepare for sleep. At san jiao time, you want to do as much as possible to help your passage.

Say a Little Prayer

The idea of saying a prayer before you get into bed is good too. I didn't have a religious upbringing but my clients who did kneel beside the bed and say things such as, 'Now I lay me down to sleep, I pray to God my soul to keep.' This is a nice thing to do to support your san jiao activities. Praying at night time puts us in the yin frame of mind for passage. It allows for our soul to journey beyond the limits of the physical world. You could also meditate to achieve this. The idea is to embrace your day with love to help support your detachment from physical references and start your journey home.

Chapter 10
Problems Solved
11 pm to 1 am

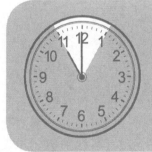

BODY PART – GALL BLAD-
DER
KEY THOUGHT – COURAGE
TIME TO . . .
Sleep, allow unconscious prob-
lem solving

COURAGE!

At 11 pm, after two hours spent in our san jiao, our chi moves to our gall bladder. We are in the time of the wood element now, which is associated with dreams, and we should be fast asleep. In fact being

Being asleep between 11 pm and 3 am, the four hours of the wood element, is crucial for health and happiness.

asleep between 11 pm and 3 am, the four hours of the wood element, is crucial for health and happiness.

Our gall bladder is associated with courage. Back in my 'perfect party day' life it was at this time of night when I had the courage to talk to people I'd been eyeing off, suggesting a dance or going somewhere more private to get to know each other. I was the lead singer in a band and it was also during gall bladder time that I could be totally outrageous on stage. But the courage the gall bladder offers is more profound and more subtle than late-night bravado. It helps us with all sorts of things in life including committing to following our dreams.

SHOULD I OR SHOULDN'T I?

It's such a waste to have lots of ideas but lack the courage to implement any of them. At some point, talking and thinking about what you want to do has to stop being theory and become reality and our gall bladder gives us the courage to make this transition.

If you are someone who has problems making decisions, small or large, it may be connected with a gall bladder deficiency. If you plan and decide, and plan and decide repeatedly it strengthens that aspect of your gall bladder. But treating your other organs well by living the chi cycle does this too. Our organs have their own special tasks but they are designed to support and help each other. The more things we do right by one organ, the better our whole system works. When the system is operating perfectly all the pieces fall into place for us to become a kind of supercomputer, capable of achieving anything.

Sleep on it

If we are asleep during gall bladder time we can actually access the universe's problem-solving service. This is why it is always best if you have a problem to 'sleep on it'. Don't try and sort it out when you are tired and overworked. It is

If we are asleep during gall bladder time we can actually access the universe's problem-solving service.

much more effective to go home, switch off at kidney time, warm your soul at pericardium time, go to bed at san jiao time, go to sleep and let your gall bladder and the universe take care of your problems. You can wake up refreshed with a new solution to what may have seemed utterly hopeless the evening before.

But this free problem-solving service won't happen if you live the day according to your own rules, then race to bed at gall bladder time. The gall bladder requires all the other actions of your day to be in harmony with the universal forces in order to offer this terrific service. You need to have gone to bed at san jiao time to receive its gift of passage, and so on, all the way back to when you got out of bed in the morning.

THE LANGUAGE OF LIFE

It is said that our organs express their unconscious selves between 11 pm and 3 am when our unconscious reigns and we dream. If you have a gall bladder deficiency you may have dreams of fights, trials and suicide. Lung deficiency generates dreams of bloody killings, war and battles. If you have dreams of forests, trees and grass it is related to your liver, as are dreams of being unable to run or move.

I think of our dreams as a universal symbolic language. Each organ is associated with different visuals and I often get these symbolic images coming to me when I take a patient's pulse prior to acupuncture treatments. Depending on which section of the wrist you use and the pressure you apply with your fingertips, you can diagnose the state of a person's organs and gain another layer of insight into what the patient is feeling.

We all have access to this symbolic language and it can provide insight and guidance for us in life. All we have to do is follow the chi cycle.

THE CLOAK OF INVISIBILITY

If we stick to the Perfect Day Plan, we will be more prone to positive emotions and actions. If you have no judgement of others, no issues with anyone, no frustration, anger, bitterness or desire for revenge, you become untouchable. If you really want to change the planet and help others, change yourself first. All you have to do is make the effort to adjust your lifestyle and think of your actions in regard to your organs.

YIN AND YANG AND INSOMNIA

Gall bladder time is when insomniacs realise they are about to have another sleepless night. Sleep is really important for health, but at the same time you need to be healthy to get a good night's sleep. The health of your gall bladder has an influence on the quality and length of sleep you get. If it is deficient, you will have trouble sleeping or wake up in the early hours and be unable to fall asleep again. Insomnia is becoming common because so many of us are unhealthy and way out of alignment with the chi cycle.

Sleep is the ultimate yin activity. But if your days are all yang, yang, yang (action, action, action) and you keep ignoring the yin (rest)

If we stick to the Perfect Day Plan, we will be more prone to positive emotions and actions. If you have no judgement of others, no issues with anyone, no frustration, anger, bitterness or desire for revenge, you become untouchable.

The health of your gall bladder has an influence on the quality and length of sleep you get. If it is deficient, you will have trouble sleeping or wake up in the early hours and be unable to fall asleep again.

times at breakfast, between 1 and 3 pm and between 5 and 9 pm, instead of drifting away when you close your eyes somewhere between 9 and 11 pm you are wired. Your bed feels like a concrete slab, you toss and turn for hours and can't fall asleep.

Drugged Sleep

People who suffer from insomnia often turn to sleeping pills to 'fix' the problem. But we humans are not machines to be fixed, we are extraordinary creations that shift all the time. Transforming things rather than fixing them is the way to go. You can't fix insomnia when you are lying awake in bed in the middle of the night. Changing your lifestyle is how you can transform insomnia into deep, peaceful sleep.

I completely understand the desire to use sleeping pills but would not recommend it as a long-term solution. In traditional Chinese medicine you are present elsewhere while you sleep and valuable work is being done on your body and spirit. Sleeping medications interfere with this and you don't recover properly from your day's activities and feel groggy and tired the next morning. Instead of experiencing a fresh start you feel as if it is just a continuation of the previous day.

Night Patrol

When I started my acupuncture business, I knew about the chi cycle but hadn't discovered how important it was to live the *whole* cycle. I didn't understand the necessity of becoming increasingly yin as the day progressed. I went along with the chi cycle up to about 3 pm but I never switched off at kidney time (5 to 7 pm) and always worked through pericardium time (7 to 9 pm). Each night it was harder to sleep. Finally it was impossible.

Some people look forward to going to bed but insomniacs dread it. I'd lie there simultaneously alert and exhausted. I tried everything to make me sleep. I'd drink wine or gulp down herbal sleeping potions, but the imbalances were so strong by then I'd end up on 'night patrol', wandering around the house in the dark. Desperate, I tried medication but felt even worse the next morning.

If you catch yourself before you go too far down that insomnia-ridden yang path, herbal sleep mixtures from naturopaths or raw herbs from practitioners of Chinese medicine can be really effective. They work with the energy systems of the body to counter an imbalanced day and prepare your body for passage—and you won't feel groggy the next morning.

My long period of insomnia made me realise that you can't just do the bits of the chi cycle that suit you. Building yin is a key part of it.

Don't Sleep In

If you are experiencing sleep disorders, try and avoid sleeping in if possible regardless of how tired you are or how little sleep you had. Sleeping in doesn't work because after a certain time your organs are not supporting sleep any more. This is why you rarely wake refreshed. You are better off making yourself get up early and getting in tune with the chi cycle. Obviously there are exceptions to this—new mothers need to sleep whenever they can and, if you are sick, spending a couple of days in bed can be healing and necessary. Generally speaking, though, sleeping in is an activity to add to your feast-day list.

THE POWER OF YIN

In our active yang culture we have all sorts of ways of measuring yang. We compete to see how many kilos we can bench press, how fast and how far we can run, or how long and how hard we can work each day. We all understand this yang because it is simple to build. What we don't understand is the power of yin.

If you want to measure the power of yin, go spend time with someone who intensely aggravates you—family members are ideal—and see how long it takes for you to blow up. The winner is the person who does not react to anything, who accepts everyone and everything the way it is.

If you want to measure the power of yin, go spend time with someone who intensely aggravates you—family members are ideal—and see how long it takes for you to blow up.

If you have yin you have the space to consider your responses. You won't react emotionally regardless of how many buttons are pushed. Yin power is priceless. Imagine a world where no one ever aggravated or annoyed you, where you didn't mind standing in queues and enjoyed being put on hold by automated phone messages. It is yin that delivers this. It allows you to wait, to really listen to people, to eat slowly enough that you can digest your food, to sleep each night, to feel peace. Balancing yang and yin makes you a better person. Think about yin power the next time you are tempted to skip breakfast, eat on the run, scream at someone or work late into the night.

CHI IN CHARGE

Shifting your day so that you get to bed in san jiao time, between 9 and 11 pm, and are then asleep during gall bladder time brings huge benefits. But if the idea of going to bed early seems totally impossible, start making small steps towards it. Everything gradually aligns itself and after a while change happens naturally. It is as if the universe picks up on your efforts and adds momentum to the process. By the time I understood that it was not a good idea to be busy all the time and work myself into the ground, I started going to bed around ten-thirty. I gradually pared this back with the ultimate goal of getting to bed by ten. As I kept building yin by respecting activities such as switching off, I found myself going to bed earlier without thinking about it. These days I'm usually asleep by nine-thirty.

I can hear you all thinking, 'In bed by nine-thirty, how boring. I'll miss my favourite TV shows, dinners out and going clubbing.' The idea is not to be rigid about going to bed early every night. Try for a few nights per week to help your organs out. You could also start making some changes to your social life by swapping some dinner dates with breakfasts or lunches. These can be even more satisfying than evening get togethers, particularly at lunchtime when our chi is in our hearts and we have the opportunity for really meaningful interactions with people.

THE PERFECT FEAST DAY

Always remember you have your feast day every week to look forward to. Make it a day of absolute indulgence. Sleep in, have sex and go for a coffee—lots of it if you want. Have a fry-up for breakfast, eat cream cakes for morning tea, toasted cheese sandwiches for lunch and more cakes and sweets for afternoon tea. Watch TV, go out for drinks and a big dinner, stay up late and watch three movies in a row. The great thing is when you don't do these things every day, you really, really enjoy them on feast day.

Of course what happens eventually is that you start feeling unwell after a feast day. That leads to a reassessment of just how important that 'treat food' is to you and what it really does. I have reached the point where I can't even tolerate sugar any more, so go for it while you can!

Following the Perfect Day Plan and getting in tune with the chi cycle is a great adventure. Don't think about it as giving up things, but as discovering new things about yourself and the universe.

Chapter 11

Restoration Time

1 am to 3 am

BODY PART – LIVER
KEY THOUGHT – RECOVER
TIME TO ...
Sleep, let your soul go home

SERIOUSLY NOW, GO TO SLEEP

At 1 am our chi moves to our liver, yet another fascinating organ. We are still under the influence of the wood element, which is connected with dreaming while we are asleep and with pursuing our dreams while awake. During the two hours of liver time we are in one of the most yin periods of the whole chi cycle, so we too should be totally yin, as in flat out and fast asleep.

GOING HOME

During the day our soul (or Hun in traditional Chinese medicine) participates in planning and direction in life (a role of the liver). While we sleep, however, our Hun leaves our body and travels to the higher planes and we can receive spiritual direction and guidance. Most of us won't remember this advice when we wake up and we are not meant to. But we are supposed to work with this material in a subconscious way during the magic hours of the metal element between 3 and 7 am.

DOPE DREAMING

This idea of our liver being connected with spiritual guidance, out-of-body travel and so on might sound a bit far-fetched, but if you have ever had one of those dreams where you have been told something you need to follow up on, or met with someone who is no longer on earth, it is connected with this aspect of the liver. Also, if you are one of the millions of people who have tried marijuana or hashish, you have had a firsthand experience of this function of the liver.

Marijuana is the most popular drug on the planet, and in my opinion this is because it enhances the functions of the liver and creates states which are connected with our true nature. We are also drawn to sugar, alcohol, caffeine and other drugs for a similar reason. They make us feel alive and energised, they break the monotony of daily life and give us a glimpse of how things could be or even how things are supposed to be.

We are drawn to sugar, alcohol, caffeine and other drugs. They make us feel alive and energised, they break the monotony of daily life and give us a glimpse of how things could be or even how things are supposed to be.

RESTORATION AND RECOVERY

We are not here to have a lifetime of boredom, stress and struggle. We are designed to have passionate, rewarding and exciting lives and, subconsciously, we know this. Challenges are a part of this, but these were intended to be tackled with healthy organs and the support of universal energy stores. The chi cycle gets our organs into shape and gets us in touch with our energy support network so that we can meet our challenges successfully.

Getting sleep in liver time is a spiritually and physically important part of this. While our heart is considered as the emperor, our liver is compared to a general because it is responsible for the overall planning of the body's functions.

Our liver regulates and stores our blood, making sure it is taken to the appropriate places at the appropriate times and giving us energy throughout the day.

While we sleep our blood returns to the liver to be cleansed and revitalised.

While we sleep our blood returns to the liver to be cleansed and revitalised. You can assist this process by sleeping in a position in which your liver is the lowest organ in the body. Ideally this is lying on your right side with your liver towards the mattress, also known as the coma or recovery position.

Women and Liver Sleep

When you wake up feeling refreshed and revitalised after a good night's sleep it is partially a result of the blood-restorative properties of liver-time sleep. Women can be particularly sensitive to the benefits of this as healthy blood and liver chi are two of the most important factors contributing to their emotional balance. The liver function of storing blood has a major influence on menstruation, too, and many gynaecological problems are connected with a malfunction of liver chi and deficient blood.

So many women are overworked and blood depleted these days that the desire to get to bed and get to sleep is often overwhelming. This contributes to the 'not tonight, dear' scenario and it is easy for their partner to feel rejected. This then affects their behaviour, which swings back to the woman who complains that 'he always want sex'. All this creates needless tension, and in no time you have a major relationship problem and it is all down to your chi and your blood.

If you have blood depletion or blood deficiency, as well as doing the things discussed in the san jiao chapter I would add in a weekly or fortnightly session of acupuncture or deep tissue massage to keep your chi and blood moving. Also, allow yourself more sleep by getting to bed earlier to benefit from the restorative properties of liver-time sleep.

Blood and Bingeing

Blood depletion leads to bingeing on sweet foods, so making sure you are asleep during gall bladder and liver time will impact on your weight as well. Sugar cravings are your body screaming out for nutrients. Things are getting serious so the organs send out an SOS. When this happens the mind conjures up an image for you to act on. In the old days this may have been a vision of a big hunk of mammoth fat; these days it is fast foods high in fat and sugar.

> Sugar cravings are your body screaming out for nutrients.

I treat a lot of kids and adults who can sit down and eat entire cakes or packets of chocolate biscuits in one session. They have serious weight problems and have been told to exercise and eat less, but the underlying issue is often nutrient and blood depletion. This prevents all your organs from working properly so you won't feel like exercising and you won't have the taste for healthy food. Tackle the depleted blood and nutrient deficiency *first*, and gradually replace some of the munchies with a healthier version. Get enough sleep. Then, once you start to feel more happy, energetic or alive, it is easier to make lifestyle changes.

HAPPY CHI

Each of our organs is associated with positive and negative emotions. Our liver is associated with happiness because it is responsible for the smooth flow and direction of chi or energy in our body, one of the things that makes us feel happy. Sugar gives the impression of enhanced chi flow, which is another reason people love it. Marijuana can also activate this chi flow. You feel so stress-free and happy you can collapse in laughter at the slightest thing. But the happiness is really coming from your chi moving freely, not from the dope or sugar.

RED EYE

Many of us are not asleep during liver time—it is common to regularly work late or party into the night. If this is the case the liver cannot do its work properly and chi cannot flow smoothly around your body, and you end up feeling grumpy and tense.

Each organ is connected with a sensory organ. Our stomach is connected with taste and our liver with our eyes. Lots of late nights and lack of sleep inhibits the liver's function of nourishing the eyes, so they become red or glassy. If you stay awake during liver time you also rob the body of an important opportunity to cleanse itself, to recover and to build immunity. So as well as feeling irritable, frustrated and gritty-eyed, you will be more prone to illness. Constant late nights eventually make you feel 'dirty' on waking up. You can also experience nausea, a bitter taste in your mouth, a lump in your throat and a general feeing of being unwell.

> Lots of late nights and lack of sleep inhibits the liver's function of nourishing the eyes, so they become red or glassy.

BUTTER FINGERS

With liver deficiencies you can end up with 'butter fingers'. In traditional Chinese medicine it is said that a healthy liver means 'the feet can walk, the hands can hold and the fingers can grasp'. If the liver is not able to work properly, it cannot regulate blood flow to the appropriate places at the appropriate times. This means things literally slip through your fingers. (In traditional Chinese medicine, Parkinson's disease is an imbalance connected with the liver.)

So when you have those days where you fumble and drop

> When you have those days where you fumble and drop everything or fall over easily, think about doing something nice for your liver.

everything or fall over easily, think about doing something nice for your liver. This means getting our day in alignment as much as possible with the chi cycle so we can go to bed during san jiao time and then have uninterrupted sleep until 3 am when our chi moves to our lungs.

NOT THE PARTY ORGAN

It is becoming harder to align ourselves with the chi cycle. Not only do we have insomnia and bad habits such as working all night, we also have a massive increase in the use of the super-intense yang stimulant drugs such as crack, ice and speed. This has a major impact on our liver-time sleep. Many people use these drugs and frequently stay up for four to six days in a row with no sleep. These drugs can accelerate organ depletion to the point where you can become seriously psychotic in a very short space of time. Getting no sleep is a major contributor to this.

Of course if you are young, staying up all night with friends is an important part of your development, but after a while it is no longer necessary. So party on, but make sure you are also identifying what dreams you want to pursue in life so that once you are done with the raging, you have a goal and know how to live the chi cycle so that you can achieve it. If you don't know how to live you will always look back at 'the good old days' and try to recapture them through drink and drugs. Once you get to your thirties or forties this is going to start drawing on your inner stores of chi, and a host of unpleasant reverse cycle symptoms will arise.

THE LAST PASSAGE

Partying is fun. I'm the first to admit that, but we are here to achieve a specific task or set of tasks, then die. We should be aiming for not only the perfect day, but the perfect death. This requires preparation, and living the chi cycle provides this in many ways.

Living your day in a way that enables you to go to bed early, fall into another dimension with san jiao passage and be fast asleep during gall bladder and liver time so that your soul can travel home is one of these. When we die we have a similar, but more amazing, experience of passage.

These days, many of us don't have a strong enough belief to support us through our final passage. We need a new set of skills. We want to be facing death with the ability to hand over, let go, make transitions. All this comes from the daily chi cycle. Following its guidelines also teaches us to trust, to understand our role in creation, and view our death as the perfect climax to our life.

Chapter 12
The Magic Hours
3 am to 5 am

BODY PART – LUNG

KEY THOUGHT – EMBODI-MENT

TIME TO . . .

Let your soul come home

RE-ENTERING THE ATMOSPHERE

At 3 am our chi leaves our liver and moves to our lungs, the organ which allowed us to take our first breath and which will usher us out with our last breath. We could think of our lungs as an intermediary between us and the visible and invisible worlds. That is why our lungs are also responsible for the return of our soul (or Hun) each morning.

At 3 am our Hun returns to the physical body, bringing lots of great information with it. Between 3 and 5 am, when our chi is in our lungs, and between 5 and 7 am, when it moves to our large intestine, is the time to process this information and embody our dreams. In lung time, however, the key to our destiny is as close as it is going to get in the next 24 hours.

SPIRIT TIME

Each night when we go to bed our passage during san jiao time dismantles us, and allows us to experience ourselves as spirit. At 3 am, as the return to our physical body takes place, a cross-over between worlds is occurring. If you are awake at this time you can consciously participate in your soul coming back to your body. This makes 3 am a prime time for serious spiritual work, which is why gurus, monks, yogis and spiritual devotees get up then to meditate.

I wouldn't start jumping out of bed and meditating at 3 am though, at least not until you've got the chi, blood and organ health to back this up. At 3 am we normal folks should still be asleep. This enables the universe, our organs and soul to go about their spiritual business in peace. But remaining asleep while our Hun re-enters the atmosphere requires yin, the one thing most of us have in short supply. We are all holding on so tight to our emotional baggage and going so fast we have trouble doing things that build yin. This makes it hard for our organs to do their job properly at those times when yin is needed, and 3 am is one of these.

Huston, we have a Problem!

The outcome of lacking yin is that lots of people automatically wake up around 3 am. This is not because they are secretly enlightened but because they don't have enough yin to support the embodiment of the soul. Our speedy yang lifestyle might be satisfying for our minds but it is creating a range of physical and spiritual imbalances. If we don't have enough yin to sleep properly we don't receive our guidance and direction and our soul can't cruise home in comfort. We can still get up the next morning and have coffee, start doing things fast, go to work and get caught up in the dramas of the day, but underneath a little cog in the big wheel is rusting. If we don't correct this, it will put pressure on other parts of our organ system. They will falter.

Soul Brothers

As well as our Hun or ethereal soul we also have what is called the Po or corporeal soul. Our Hun and Po work together; the Hun is connected with our dreams in life and the Po helps us make them a reality. Traditional Chinese medicine is extraordinary and mystical as well as practical, simple yet profound. It covers every aspect of our lives from the functioning of the visible parts to the invisible parts, our spirit and soul. This is a system so intelligent it beggars belief. Even though we can't see our soul or what it gets up to while we sleep, if we follow the Perfect Day Plan we can rest assured that everything is being taken care of and everything is unfolding as it should.

MISSION ACCEPTED

If we sleep during gall bladder and liver time, between 11 pm and 3 am, we can benefit from the travels of our soul, and the subconscious planning and decision-making of our gall bladder and liver. This is when we receive our mission for the day ahead. Our job is to accept that mission each morning during lung or large intestine time by waking up in the time of the metal element and getting into our bodies rather than our heads. This means our organs can carry out their tasks, and we can achieve our destiny.

Po is connected with our lungs and breath. Our lungs assist our heart in controlling blood circulation. Our blood, an elixir of life, holds the information our soul received while we slept. If we get up and do some exercise, we engage our lungs and activate blood circulation. This in turn circulates our soul's instructions throughout our body. Every organ receives that information, so every organ knows exactly what they have to do with it to make it real.

THE DREAM MACHINE

Some people recommend having a notebook and pen by the bed so that when you wake, the first thing you do is write down what you remember of your dreams. Apparently you have about thirty seconds before the memories are gone. But instead of trying to get this down on paper and deciphering its meaning, I would get straight into Chi-gung (see p. 151) and exercise. This allows you to interpret your dreams by engaging body, mind, breath, chi, blood and spirit. It is a much more effective way of working with that information.

> Instead of trying to get this down on paper and deciphering its meaning, get straight into Chi-gung and exercise.

This is how our dreams are supposed to be interpreted. Writing them down and analysing them is *theoretical*. If you start writing the moment you get out of bed, it is easy to add a cup of coffee and then before you know it you are into the stress of the day and another opportunity for your body and for building yin slips past. Our minds are already having way too much fun and getting all the attention. They can be let off the leash later at spleen time, between 9 and 11 am, when there is full backing for them to roam free.

THE TREASURE CHEST

In the time of the lungs we want to be in our bodies. Like all our organs, our lungs have many roles. They inhale pure chi and exhale toxic chi so they play a role in 'letting go' and embracing the new. If we have healthy lung chi we have warm hands, we breathe easily and our sense of smell is normal. Weak lung chi means we have cold limbs and hands. It can also cause accumulation of chi in the chest, so you get coughing, stuffiness and breathlessness.

We want strong lung chi and not just so we have a nice warm handshake. With strong lung chi we are able to live in the now, accept the past and look forward to the future. Imagine simply not caring about anything that happened to you, being absolutely free of concern about anything anyone had ever said to you or about you in the past, regardless of how hurtful it was. Imagine being so present all the time you never drag up old arguments in your head and re-run them. This is what our lungs are designed to deliver.

> With strong lung chi we are able to live in the now, accept the past and look forward to the future.

The Inner Glow

Our chest is called the 'sea of chi'. Our lungs spread this treasure throughout our body to help all the organs function. They also spread body fluids to the skin in the form of a fine 'mist'. This protects us. As our lungs circulate blood and chi, they nourish our skin and hair.

> As our lungs circulate blood and chi, they nourish our skin and hair.

Do something nice for your lungs, and by default every other organ, by following the Perfect Day Plan and taking up the chi cycle. In return you get fresh chi, your skin and hair shine, you radiate happiness, you accept everyone, you forgive everything, you have fantastic relationships and, if you add good nutritional supplements to the mix, you have the inner glow that everyone wants.

Soul Surgery

By adding Chinese herbs and acupuncture treatments to your life, you can accelerate your path to perfect health and happiness. This is all part of the plan. Herbs and acupuncture work *with* your organs and chi; they are there to support your journey. Acupuncture keeps the energy pathways in the body free so that your chi can flow to all your organs. It treats the physical and emotional aspects of the organs, and your spirit and soul as well.

Our corporeal soul or Po is also described as the breath of life. Sadness or grief constrains Po and obstructs its movements, which is why, for example, depressed people have shallow breathing. Even though Po is part of our soul, there are lung and Po acupuncture points that have a powerful releasing effect on constrained emotions and 'firm Po'. You have to love this ancient form of medicine that can treat your soul as well as your body.

The idea is to work with everything at your disposal to build your chi, blood and yin and seek balance. Lung time is another part of the day where we have seen that we need more yin (rest), but this doesn't mean yang (action) is a bad thing. The nature of the universe is yang, it is ever-expanding. Because we are a part of this it is our nature and our destiny to expand too. By humankind developing and expanding our minds over the centuries we laid the foundations for a magnificent future. But along the way we forgot all about our bodies, our organs. If we now follow the Perfect Day Plan and use the chi cycle to bring our bodies up to the speed of our minds, we will be on the track to destiny. The next two hours, as our chi moves to our large intestine, is when we put the last piece of the puzzle in place for this.

Chapter 13

Ready For a Brand New Day

5 am to 7 am

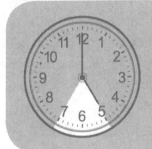

BODY PART – LARGE INTESTINE
KEY THOUGHT – TRANSFORM
TIME TO . . .
Wake up and start a perfect day

WAKING UP WITH THE WORLD

At 5 am our chi or inner energy moves to our large intestine. This is another organ connected with 'letting go' physically and emotionally, so each morning between 5 and 7 am is the best time to get rid of all our old crap and start afresh. It is the best time of the entire 24 hours to transform ourselves.

Between 5 and 7 am we are in the time of the metal element so we have an opportunity to 'wake with the sword in hand'. We can cut out what we no longer want, vanquish our inner demons and win the battles that will help change our lives. After 7 am this opportunity is gone, so the most important thing to do in large intestine time is to get up as close to five as possible.

Most people hate the idea of getting up early. My clients will frequently say 'I'm not a morning person' but we were all originally 'morning people'—it is just that by the time we grow up we have picked up lots of bad habits. We stay up late, skip meals, sleep in, eat junk food, get really stressed and don't switch off in the evening. All these habits make it harder to go to bed, harder to get a good night's sleep and really tough to get up early the following morning. So, you wake up, you might have every intention of getting up, but your eyes are heavy, your bed pulls you back in, and before you know it you are asleep again. This will not be quality sleep though and you won't feel better for it when you eventually do get up. To combat this, make yourself sit up as soon as you wake, drink some water and get away from the bed as fast as possible. Splash some water on your face and chest to wake yourself up.

> People often tell me they don't want to get up early because they love their beds and their sleep. If this is the case, go to bed earlier and really enjoy it.

People often tell me they don't want to get up early because they love their beds and their sleep. If this is the case, go to bed earlier and really enjoy it. If that doesn't sound appealing, it usually means you don't love your bed, rather you hate facing the discomfort of getting up. If we let this discomfort rule us, we will never discover the potential of the day or get the wisdom, courage, support, joy, purpose and other fabulous things on offer.

The more we bring our lifestyles into alignment with the chi cycle, the more we benefit from the forces of yin and yang and the easier it is to become 'morning people' and start a new life of increasing energy and vitality. Getting up with the birds is fantastic. There's nothing like the smell of potential in the morning. Simply stepping outside and feeling the excitement and energy of a brand new day is a great thing to do. If you want to achieve your dreams it is an *essential* thing to do. If you want to be happy, healthy and successful there are a few things that are non-negotiable, and getting up early is one of them. So, if you can only change one thing in your life, make it getting up earlier.

If you want to be happy, healthy and successful there are a few things that are non-negotiable, and getting up early is one of them.

SIT AND DELIVER

Once you are up, one of the first things to do is to have a bowel movement. The time between 5 and 7 am is all about letting go, and faeces is simply an accumulation of old stuff that has been digested, processed and is now ready to be eliminated. Drink a couple of glasses of water to help trigger the elimination process. Then sit on the toilet. Even if you don't manage to pass anything it helps get the habit in place.

In traditional Chinese medicine your bowel movements are really important. In ancient times, the texture, colour, smell and frequency of a person's motions were key indicators of the health of their organs. Although not many of us want to revive that particular art form, generally speaking your stool should be nice and soft and well-formed. Ideally, we would have bowel movements twice a day. Less than once a day is constipation, and can lead towards serious illness. After seven days without a bowel movement the levels of toxins that have built up in your body can kill you.

Hang On

Regular bowel movements are crucial to your health and happiness. If we don't have a bowel movement before seven in the morning, we start the day with a toxin build-up.

So, regular bowel movements are crucial to your health and happiness. If we don't have a bowel movement before seven in the morning, we start the day with a toxin build-up. This means we start with a physical and emotional handicap, feeling stuck and out of sorts. Because of our diet and our reverse cycle lifestyle, constipation is common. I treat many clients whose bowels only move twice a week.

For westerners it takes around three days from eating something to it leaving our body as stool. Even then we don't pass everything we've eaten. This reflects how we are approaching life. We hang on to the past and can't let go of things. We become consumed by anger, resentment, stress and negative thoughts—we live in a state of resistance. We don't do this deliberately; it is because we have forgotten how else we can live.

Let Go

Wellness and inspirational books are always suggesting we 'let go' or 'go with the flow'. People tend to interpret 'letting go' as a state of mind, but it is also to do with our body— our organs and chi. It's hard to let go on any level if you feel unsafe and, as we have seen, due to our depleted organs and blood many of us feel this way. Once we get back in tune with the chi cycle, we build up our inner resources and we begin to feel our connection with the life forces again. Then we automatically start to relax and let go. Chi can flow through us in harmony with the natural forces. This improves bowel function as well, as constipation is the absence of the wavelike movements that keep our bowels moving.

FLEXIBLE BODY/FLEXIBLE MIND

When we have a bowel movement, it physically empties the old stuff. But in large intestine time we have the chance to do the same emotionally. When we wake up, around 95 per cent of our thoughts are going to be from the past. If you lie in bed and let your mind go, it will instantly start to replay things that happened yesterday, the day before, or even weeks or months before. This could be a rehashing of arguments, or re-living work or family dramas. But right now, between 5 and 7 am, we have full support to clear out as much of this as possible so we don't have to lug it around for another day.

Being flexible is important. If your body is not flexible, your mind is not flexible and change will be out of the question. So once you are up and about, do some stretching to increase your flexibility. Reach your arms up to the ceiling, reach down towards your toes a couple of times. Do some side stretches. Certain stretches activate certain organs and meridians, improve their function and help your chi to flow.

Meditate

Each of our organs supports a certain action and a certain way of thinking. Large intestine time has the dual function of letting go of the old and bringing in the new. This means between 5 and 7 am you have full universal support to break free from your limiting thought patterns and embrace a new way of thinking. Seeing how meditation is all about letting go of the old and receiving the new, it makes meditation a perfect large intestine time activity. Particularly in that first hour, between 5 and 6 am, when you also have easy access to the universal intelligence, Tao or mind of God. It is definitely

Between 5 and 7 am you have full universal support to break free from your limiting thought patterns and embrace a new way of thinking.

the best time of day to meditate (apart from 3 am for the advanced meditators), as later in the day it is more difficult and far less effective.

Still Your Mind

A lot of people think that meditation is about sitting and trying to still your mind. But our minds are naturally expansive and yang. It takes years to learn to control them and we just don't have that kind of time any more. As speedy yang people we need a form of meditation that, like sex, engages all our senses so that the mind naturally stills. During sex you don't have to focus on controlling your mind because, as the intensity of the experience increases, thoughts become totally single-minded until the orgasmic unification of mind and body occurs.

I practise and teach a form of meditation that creates a similar state of body–mind unification. You don't have to focus on stilling the mind because the experience is so overwhelming, it happens naturally. This technique is not connected with any particular doctrine or belief system. There are many of these powerful new forms of meditation around now but, unlike relaxation techniques which many people confuse with meditation, you need someone to teach you.

The Chi of Weight Loss

Between 5 and 7 am is the very best time of the day to exercise. It might feel easier later in the day when we are less emotionally vulnerable and more flexible, which is why lots of people go to the gym after work, but morning is the time to do it. This is not only because exercise is another activity which can transform the old into the new, but because of its impact on controlling weight. Physical activity increases the rate at which your body burns fat. If you exercise early in the morning on an empty stomach, it burns fat 300 times faster than if you do it in the evening. I have worked with numerous clients who exercised after work for years and never got the results they wanted, but once they switched to early morning sessions they noticed dramatic changes within weeks.

> If you exercise early in the morning on an empty stomach, it burns fat 300 times faster than if you do it in the evening.

It's Elemental

The metal element is like the blade that cuts wood; wood is connected to the liver and the liver regulates the release of fat deposits. So from both east and west perspectives, you are best off exercising in the morning. It stabilises your emotions, reduces your cravings and increases your energy. It makes following the rest of the day's chi cycle easier. It also allows you to develop deeper breathing and it contributes to healthy bowel movements. All these things mean weight loss will happen naturally.

Transformational Exercises

I wouldn't exercise at large intestine time just to lose weight—it has way more potential than this. You can use it to convert negative emotions into positive—the old into the new. You see, our emotions are stored in our muscles and when we do repetitive movements these emotions can be released. A lot of runners experience this. There they are jogging along minding their own business, when suddenly they start having angry thoughts about people or flashbacks to old hurts and insults. Not understanding why this happens, they get stuck in long arguments in their heads with the offending person. This is a release of old emotional stuff, and once it comes forward you can take the opportunity to let it go rather than cement it in.

If you want to get into processing negative emotions in this way but don't like to run, cycling is also good. Any form of endurance exercise that you almost dread doing, where within minutes your mind will automatically be suggesting you stop, is the right psychological environment for transformation. Lots of people go to the gym or run on a treadmill and zone out by watching TV or listening to music, or they hire a personal trainer who chats non-stop about new recipes or what they did on the weekend. This is a good way to break into exercising and it is a great work-out for the physical body, but if we are making the effort to exercise we might as well get the most out of it and use it to improve ourselves emotionally as well.

MUSCLE MAGIC

I am a great advocate for doing some weights in large intestine time. People tend to resist the idea of weights because they think it means standing in a gym in skimpy shorts and admiring yourself in a mirror. The first thing I have to ask is: what is wrong with that? Our bodies are fantastic and amazing, and if you have spent a lot of time and effort working on your body of course you should admire the outcome. Even if we haven't worked on our bodies, we should all be able to stand in front of a mirror and admire ourselves, rather than obsessing over our flaws. Having said that, you can easily injure yourself when using weights so it is important to be aware of what you are doing all the time. Working with a mirror keeps you focused. It also allows you to physically project your goals.

Weights: The Yoga of the West

Using weights is not body building, it is about building muscle. Weights are sometimes called the 'yoga of the west' and this is absolutely true. Doing weights breaks down muscle fibre and rebuilds stronger fibres. As your emotions are stored in your muscles, this is an incredible opportunity to break down stored memories and emotions, and entrenched ideas as well. As we rebuild muscle we build powerful new thought programs of ourselves as happy, healthy and successful.

Many 'psychological' problems can be tackled through the body. If you have certain issues like back pain, which relates to 'carrying the load', and are conscious of this in your exercise program, you can work with it and save a fortune in therapists' fees!

The upper half of the body is all about emotions. If you do some chest presses you will

Many 'psychological' problems can be tackled through the body. The upper half of the body is all about emotions. If you do some chest presses you will immediately feel 'pumped up' physically and emotionally.

immediately feel 'pumped up' physically and emotionally. The lower half of the body is about karma. The lower body exercises are the ones many people dread. I call my squats Dr Quad because it is through them that I work with anger, frustration and family issues. I pick up heavy hand weights and slowly squat down to the ground; as I rise up I inhale and feel the muscles burn. I visualise all those negative emotions burning with it.

The Power of Weights

Weights-work is right in tune with the morning's transformational theme because if you understand its potential you can make yourself into anything. I remember an old interview with Arnold Schwarzenegger, when he was only known in body-building circles. He was asked what he was going to do with his future. In my memory he said he was going to be a politician. The interviewer resisted the impulse to laugh in his face, as Arnie was quite big and scary-looking, and then asked him how he was going to do that. 'I'm going to keep pushing my weights,' Arnie replied, and the rest, as they say, is history.

SAY CHI

Between 5 and 7 am is also the best time to get to know our chi. It's one of the three treasures of Chinese medicine that, if nurtured, deliver health, happiness and success. We have our own chi or energy in our body, but to be operating at our full potential and getting all the great gifts of the chi cycle we need to build and replenish this at every opportunity. The universe has a limitless supply and if we live in harmony with the cycle and do chi work, we can tap into this.

Chi-gung introduces us to our chi and shows how to access it from the universal stores. The next step is to learn how to move that energy, and this is where Tai-chi comes in. It teaches us to move chi around our body but also how to make transitions from being yang to being yin. This is an invaluable skill for 21st century super yang people. If we know what shifting from yang to yin feels like, we can draw upon that feeling later in the day at breakfast time, lunchtime and after work when we need to switch from one to the other. As we have seen, our health, happiness and maybe even our lives depend on our ability to do this. (Tai-chi and Chi-gung are powerful anti-ageing tools as well!)

So do yourself a really big favour and take up some chi classes. Most are offered in the evening, as the teachers are probably doing their chi practice in the morning. I suggest learning the moves in lessons whenever you can, but focus on doing chi work in the morning when you have best access to universal chi stores.

WAKING WITH THE SWORD IN HAND

Getting up, exercising and building your chi might sound like a lot of things to do in only two hours, but I have condensed it into an accelerated program where the total time per week is only seven hours. When you consider that most people spend on average up to forty hours per week watching TV, reshuffling things and taking seven of those hours to do some self-transformation is possible.

I meditate and do Tai-chi and Chi-gung every day and then alternate weights one day with endurance exercise, such as running or working on a cross-trainer, on another. Five to 7 am is the crucial part of the day for me. In those two hours I get what I need to achieve all my goals, physical and emotional. Large intestine time is the only chance each day to grasp the sword and make the big changes, so grab it while you can. The rewards are beyond belief.

Morning Glory

> Many men naturally wake with an erection, but this does not mean it is time to have sex.

For men there's another version of 'waking with the sword in hand', the infamous 'morning glory'. Many men naturally wake with an erection, but this does not mean it is time to have sex. If you do you won't want to get out of bed, let alone do chi work and exercise. If you don't believe me give it a go and see how you feel.

The chi cycle is all about learning to work with our chi or energy intelligently. There are times of the day to build, share or conserve energy. Now, between 5 and 7 am, is the time for *building* chi. Unfortunately, you can't do this by having sex in the morning. However, as we have seen, there is lots of time later on for sex, from 5 pm in kidney time and onwards is ideal—it will be more satisfying then and also more beneficial. Don't sleep through these two hours of large intestine time either, because sleeping between 5 and 7 am doesn't build chi. That happens when you sleep between 10 pm and 3 am.

THE STOCKPILE

While we are on the subject of 'don't do's', try and avoid coffee and cigarettes in large intestine time too. If you have been living the reverse cycle by sleeping in, struggling towards caffeine to wake you up, working hard, eating poorly, staying up late, suffering sleep disorders, stressing out then starting that all over again the next day, a lot of physical and emotional toxins build up. You don't notice this while you are asleep, because everything is effortless, but when you wake up reality hits and things don't look or feel too good. Coffee or cigarettes appear to improve the situation because they create the impression of chi or energy moving. The problem is, those underlying negative emotions and imbalances won't go away on their own—you have to make them.

The universe is going to support you doing this each morning. To make the process easier, as soon as you wake up it lays out a smorgasbord of things you don't want to be or feel. This is an opportunity for you to go through and sweep what you don't want off the table. Go for it! Out with the old and in with the new.

If you have a coffee or cigarette, or turn the TV on or do other non-transformational things, the table gets wheeled away untouched. The next morning it will be back, but with another day's worth of toxins added to your stockpile. Once the pile reaches a certain size, we enter banquet territory and it is hard to know where to even begin. It seems easier to give up and get medicated for the uncomfortable symptoms this stuff is now generating. Medication magically makes the table disappear, but the truth is it hasn't really gone anywhere. The table is waiting for you when you get off the medication, or when you die. So, instead of having a cup of coffee or a cigarette to override early morning discomfort, get into exercise or chi work instead and make your life fantastic, energetic and exciting.

Cigarettes and the Breakfast of Champions

I knew this businessman who got up each morning at five-thirty, made himself a pot of coffee, then sat down and drank two coffees and smoked three cigarettes. 'The breakfast of champions' he called it, as it would get his bowels and his mind moving for the day.

This is another example of how we can subconsciously perform actions in alignment with the chi cycle. In traditional Chinese medicine, coffee and cigarettes engage with our lungs and their partner organ, our large intestine. These are the metal element organs, the instruments of change. Cigarettes engage the lungs in particular, which are responsible for accepting the past, living in the now and embracing the future. Waking up and reaching for a ciggie does deal with the negative feelings that surface because it creates a feeling of acceptance of the moment.

Because cigarettes also engage our large intestine, which is to do with 'letting go', they can trigger a bowel movement. Coffee can do this too. But in order to do so, it does other things too like stopping the absorption of vital nutrients and reducing your appetite for food and for life. Accepting the past, embracing the future and moving our bowels are all ideal goals for 5 to 7 am, but cigarettes and coffee are not the ideal method to achieve them. This doesn't mean you have to give up your coffee or cigarettes, just have them later on, after breakfast.

THE ART OF CHANGE

Living the chi cycle is all about rescheduling things or making small changes, not focusing on giving things up.

The big changes follow the small ones and along the way you naturally lose interest in habits such as smoking. The chi cycle gives the cigarettes up for you.

When I do my workshops on the Perfect Day Plan, everyone tends to get fired up. The following morning, instead of sleeping in then heading for a coffee as they would normally do, they jump out of bed at first light, gulp down litres of water, stretch and then exercise as if their life depended on it. By the end of the week they are a wreck and return to their old lifestyle. Just as we fall off the chi cycle gradually, we want to get back on it *gradually*. If your lifestyle is way out of alignment, pace yourself. Don't suddenly shift from getting up at 8 am to getting up at 5 am. Reduce it slowly. There is an art to change.

The Time for Change

A 40-year-old guy, Mark, came to see me recently. He had started a real estate business in his early twenties. As it became more successful he had less time, so he started eating all his meals out. He always worked late to try and get on top of things. Not surprisingly he became permanently fatigued, slept in each morning, gained weight, developed high blood pressure and was then put on medication. He had serious constipation. He hated his life and his body, but most of all he hated the mornings. Getting out of bed was so hard he had to put loud alarm clocks in other rooms to make him have to get out of bed to turn them off. Then he went straight to coffee and cigarettes.

Emotionally, he was stuck in the past, irritable and easily aggravated, and frequently caught up in endless arguments in his head with family members whom he believed had wronged him in the past. He had lived like this for nearly twenty years. He was carrying an incredible accumulation of physical and emotional toxins. Each day he missed the opportunity to clear out the old and start anew so the baggage just kept piling up.

Mark said he really wanted to change and take up the chi-cycle lifestyle, but was going to wait until he had his business under control and had more time. I often hear comments like this. It might be when someone's job changes, when summer comes, when they give up smoking or when the kids leave home and so on. But there will never be the perfect circumstances for change. You have to change your internal

But there will never be the perfect circumstances for change. You have to change your internal circumstances by getting in line with the chi cycle, and then the external changes accordingly. So, in fact, it is always the right time to change.

circumstances by getting in line with the chi cycle, and then the external changes accordingly. So, in fact, it is always the right time to change.

Mark also said he felt he was too far gone to change. Even if he could get up earlier, his weight prevented him from exercising. He had been really fit when he was younger and was into weights and martial arts but now walking was a major effort. He couldn't believe what he'd done to himself. But we are not born in a culture that understands chi, so we have no idea how to live. We deplete our blood, organs and energy without knowing anything about it. We can't blame ourselves for what we don't know. Once we do know, making small changes is the key to big change.

Changing our diet is an essential part of this. Most of the food we consume is processed. It is no longer delivering us nutrients and much of it is actually costing us nutrients and chi. For Mark, I began with making adjustments to his diet. I also recommended an intensive treatment of Chinese raw herbs, nutritional supplements and the new superfoods such as the acai berry and other powerful plant-based products. I am a big fan of protein powders as well, which were developed for people wanting to reach high levels of physical performance. With our yin-deficient, protein-deficient lifestyle, we would be crazy not to take advantage of them. When this started to have an effect on Mark and his energy levels dramatically increased, we looked at knocking five minutes off the alarm clock per week. Next came some Tai-chi before coffee. A couple of months later he took up cycling for endurance training. He felt better every day.

CHI IS THE KEY

Once you get a morning routine of this sort in place and start feeling different, after a while you can't not do it. You automatically wake up early and enjoy getting into your body and feeling your chi. You look forward to your porridge and arriving. You love working productively in the morning and naturally want a wholesome nutritious lunch because you crave the way these things make you feel. The deal sweetener is your relationship improves, your sex life improves, your skin and hair improve. Your soul flourishes.

Chi is the key to it all. So, Chi-gung or Tai-chi is the first thing to take up and the one thing to never give up. As you become older or if you are not well or not fit enough for weights and strenuous exercise in the morning, the idea is to focus mainly on chi work. Regular practice keeps your body and mind flexible and you won't have an old age characterised by fear and restriction (that comes from not knowing how to live).

Chi and the Law of Attraction

There is another benefit from living the chi cycle and it is connected with the law of attraction. The law of attraction is real, but the most important aspect of making it work is *feeling* it. It is very hard to feel happy, wealthy or successful when you are annoyed, frustrated, sick, unhappy and lost. You need to *live* the chi cycle to make the law of attraction work for you, because it will let you feel positive and powerful and then you will attract.

> You need to *live* the chi cycle to make the law of attraction work for you, because it will let you feel positive and powerful and then you will attract.

Doing Chi-gung is a crucial part of this. After a while you learn how to gather chi from the universe and direct it into your body. You know what is out there for you and how powerful your ability is to attract whatever you want. There is no doubt. There's no need to talk about whether it works or not, or why it works. You *know* it works because you can feel it.

Trippy Chi

If you really get into it and do enough Chi-gung and add in meditation—the last on the list of things to add to the morning routine—you start to get amazing inter-dimensional experiences as well. Things like TV, which are not really of any benefit to us, become less interesting. Once we understand that we are chi and that everything in the universe is chi, and that we can work with that chi, all the doors of potential fly open for us.

Once we understand that we are chi and that everything in the universe is chi, and that we can work with that chi, all the doors of potential fly open for us.

Chapter 14

Living the Chi Cycle

THE EASY WAY AND THE HARD WAY

There are two ways to do life. There is the easy way, which is following the chi cycle through the Perfect Day Plan and making the most of what is already at your disposal, and the hard way, which is making up your own rules to live by. The funny thing is the easy way looks hard, and the hard way looks easy. Sleeping in each morning, using stimulants to get yourself going, eating fast food and working late at night feels easy. But the outcome is constant depletion of your blood and chi. Your health and happiness will slowly decrease and once that goes, believe me, life gets really hard. Personally I'd rather break rocks in the hot sun all day than go there.

Following the chi cycle is easy because it is what we are designed to do. Everything feels right as you do it and you feel healthier, happier and more emotionally balanced each day. While it may look hard to some, the only challenging part is getting up early and doing some Chi-gung, stretching and exercise. And of that, only the endurance exercise is hard, but in a good way. After several months even this becomes something you look forward to. The rest of it, eating a nice cooked lunch with friends, going home from work and switching off at a reasonable hour, reading a book, playing with your kids or going to bed early, isn't hard work.

You Can Take It With You

So if the idea of being happy, healthy and successful, and achieving your dreams and having great relationships isn't enough motivation to follow the chi cycle, what about this: every action we perform in harmony with our organs and the universal forces allows our organs to generate positive emotions. This affects how we live our life and interact with others. We are more likely to be loving and forgiving and understanding of others if we are healthy and happy. And, we can take all this good work with us when we go.

We are here on business and that business is self-development. We need to keep this in mind and never turn back from a challenge whether physical, emotional or spiritual. If we follow the chi cycle we are more likely to meet our challenges and achieve our goals. When we die all this work comes with us via our Hun, our soul messenger. The last thing we want to do is die, mosey over to the other side, then realise what we didn't do. We are the ones lucky enough to score a body this time round, so let's do the right thing and work with it.

The Big Picture

I really think we have no choice but to follow the Perfect Day Plan. Our 21st-century lifestyle is generating so many illnesses and imbalances that it is not sustainable—it wastes our chi. But if you live in a way that builds chi instead, each organ will become progressively more healthy. All your emotions will become more positive. As your liver chi improves you will feel happy. As your spleen chi improves you will know who you are and what your boundaries are. As your kidney chi improves so does your willpower and strength. As your lung chi improves you live in the present. If your heart chi is strong you are filled with love for yourself, your fellow humans and every living thing on the planet. You will rediscover the joy of life and you will understand your purpose here.

THE CHI CYCLE

7 am to 9 am	Stomach	Arrive	Be sweet to yourself, eat breakfast, feel balance
9 am to 11 am	Spleen	Action	Work hard, think, do
11 am to 1 pm	Heart	Love	Work smart, access your soul, spread the love
1 pm to 3 pm	Small intestine	Slow	Have lunch, go slow, ride the wave
3 pm to 5 pm	Bladder	Support	Put cruise control on, go with the flow, feel the power
5 pm to 7 pm	Kidneys	Switch off	Acknowledge strength and skills, have sex, share a laugh